AF564797

Poultry Production and Marketing

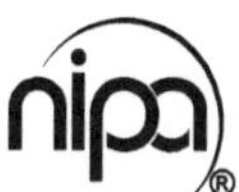

NIPA® GENX ELECTRONIC RESOURCES & SOLUTIONS P. LTD.
New Delhi-110 034

Poultry Production and Marketing

F.P. Savaliya
Principal Scientist & Head
Poultry Research Station
AAU and Core Co-PI, NAHEP-CAAST
Anand Agricultural University, Anand, Gujarat

Rais M. Rajpura
Assistant Professor & Head
Department of Animal Science
B.A. College of Agriculture
AAU and Co-PI, NAHEP-CAAST
Anand Agricultural University, Anand, Gujarat

Shakti Ranjan Panigrahy
Assistant Professor and Head
Department of Operations Management
IABMI, AAU and Co-PI, Co-PI, NAHEP- CAAST
Anand Agricultural University, Anand, Gujarat

Dilip R. Vahoniya
Assistant Professor and Head
Department of Agri Entrepreneurship and Project Management
IABMI, AAU and Co-PI, Co-PI, NAHEP- CAAST
Anand Agricultural University
Anand, Gujarat

Ashish B. Mahera
Assistant Professor and Head
Department of Marketing Management
IABMI, AAU and Co-PI, Co-PI, NAHEP- CAAST
Anand Agricultural University, Anand, Gujarat

R.S. Pundir
Principal and Dean
IABMI, AAU and Principal Investigator, NAHEP
Anand Agricultural University
Anand, Gujarat

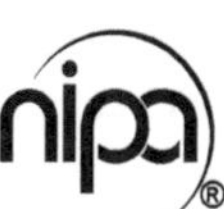

NIPA® GENX ELECTRONIC RESOURCES & SOLUTIONS P. LTD.
New Delhi-110 034

NIPA® GENX ELECTRONIC RESOURCES & SOLUTIONS P. LTD.

101,103, Vikas Surya Plaza, CU Block
L.S.C.Market, Pitam Pura, New Delhi-110 034
Ph : +91 11 4386 0225, 9717133558, 9540816132
E-mail: newindiapublishingagency@gmail.com
Website: www.nipareresources.com

Print ISBN: 978-93-58874-78-5

ebook ISBN: 978-93-58875-34-8

Composed and Designed by NIPA®.

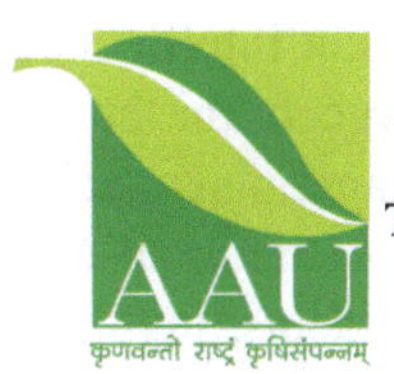

ANAND AGRICULTURAL UNIVERSITY
ANAND-388 110, GUJARAT
Tel.: (O) +91-2692-261273, Fax : (O) +91-2692-261520
Email : vc@aau.in

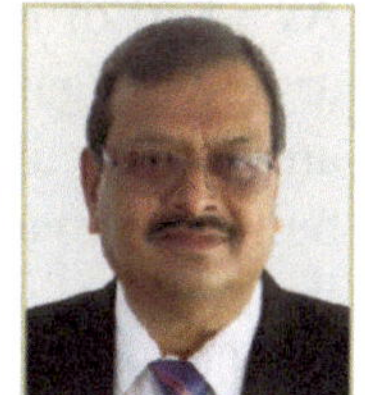

Dr. K.B. Kathiria
Vice Chancellor

Message

Agriculture is backbone of the Indian economy as, inter alia, it provides livelihood to nearly half of the country's workforce. As a result of technological advancement, enabling policy environment and hard work of farming community the country has not only become self sufficient in production of most of the crops and allied activities but also has made significant strides in the export of some Agricultural commodities. There is no denying the fact that focus in agriculture, since the time of green revolution, has been centric to production technologies.

Marketing, the key problem of farmers has not received adequate attention. Agriculture market intelligence an integral part of marketing becomes important and crucial when more than 80 per cent of the farmers in the country, who are small and marginal and constitute core production system, hardly understand the market dynamics. In view of this, there is dire need of rigorous research on various aspects of agricultural marketing with focused attention on market intelligence accompanied with capacity building of PG students, faculties, policy makers and farmers. This may go a long way in improving the existing level of higher education and eventually helping farmers to increase their income.

The Indian Council of Agricultural Research, New Delhi, with the active support of the World Bank has formulated a National Agricultural Higher Education Project (NAHEP), for improving the level of agricultural education and research in the country. In view of this, Center for Agricultural Market Intelligence under Center for Advanced Science and Technology (CAAST) component of NAHEP has been awarded to Anand Agricultural University through a competitive selection process.

As a part of its basic objective the center for agriculture market intelligence at AAU is gainfully engaged in, inter alia, conducting research in the broad area of agriculture marketing and market intelligence and organizing capacity building programmes, online and offline, involving experts of national and international repute for various stakeholders including PG students, faculties and farmers.

I am happy to know that the center has been rated top performer in the category of second phase by the World Bank and ICAR in its mid-term review meeting. I am sure the center will not only achieve its objectives under NAHEP-CAAST but also scale new heights in the time to come.

I congratulate the whole NAHEP CAAST team consisting of faculties, research staff, in general, and members of the research team, in particular of 10 commodity reports covering Wheat, Maize, Groundnut, Cumin, Potato, Poultry, Fisheries, Dairy and Food Processing. I also hope that these commodity reports will be useful for stakeholders, researchers, policy makers and all those interested in the broad area of agriculture market intelligence including allied fields.

Date : 26/04/2021 **(K.B. Kathiria)**

Preface

Anand Agricultural University has awarded an ICAR-World Bank funded project To Establish Centre for Agricultural Market Intelligence at its campus. The project is multidisciplinary project, covering crops, dairy, food processing, poultry and fisheries. The project has been sanctioned under National Agricultural Higher Education Project of the Indian Council of Agriculture Research. The major objectives of this project include price forecasting and behaviors, export competitiveness, evaluation of e-National Agri- culture Market (e-NAM), market institutions and capacity building of faculty, students, farmers and other stake holders.

Poultry sector is one of the fastest growing segments in the agricultural sector to- day with an average growth rate of 6 to 8 percent per annum. India's estimated production for the year 2018-19 was 103.3 billion numbers eggs and 4.06 million tonnes of poultry meat. The sector contributes Rs.1347.57 billion which holds 12.91 percent share in the total output of the livestock sector. It provided direct employment to 40 lakh and indirect employment to 2.5 crore people. The poultry sector in India has experienced a revolu- tionary shift in structure and operation, which has led its transformation from a simple backyard activity to a major commercial agro-based industry over a period of decades. The constant efforts in the up-gradation, modification and application of new technolo- gies lead towards the diversified and overall growth in poultry and allied sectors. Andhra Pradesh, Tamil Nadu, Telangana, and West Bengal are major producers of eggs whereas; Maharashtra, Haryana, West Bengal, Tamil Nadu, and Andhra Pradesh are the leading poultry meat-producing states in India.

In this status report, we have included topics from the history of the poultry sector to the current development of the sector. We have discussed the contribution of different components of the sector at the world, national and regional levels. Other than this, important issues like marketing, trade, government policies, challenges, and the impact of COVID-19 on the poultry sector are also included.

There are 15 chapters in this report. They are structured in such a way that all the stakeholders of the sector can take benefit from this report

NAHEP-CAAST, AAU, Anand **Authors**

Acknowledgement

The 'Centre for Agricultural Market Intelligence' under NAHEP-CAAST at AAU, Anand is comprehensive and encompasses all crucial issues, including demand-supply predictions, price forecasting, and capacity building of various stakeholders with a focus on PG students and faculties. This project is a collaborative endeavor from ICAR-World Bank, and we acknowledge the technical and financial support received from ICAR- NAHEP and World Bank.

This book is prepared by research teams mainly using time series data apart from discussions and valuable suggestions from the experts in the broad area of Agriculture and Agricultural Marketing. The book contains comprehensive observations and findings emanated from the analysis using the best available data and appropriate analytical tools. We expect that this publication will be helpful to all the concerned stakeholders, including P.G. students, researchers, and policymakers.

We are immensely indebted to Dr. R.C. Agrawal, DDG (Edu.) & National Director NAHEP, ICAR, New Delhi, for continuously enlightening us with his valuable guidance, direction, stewardship, and excellent support in the overall implementation of the project, as also bringing out this publication.

We are highly thankful to our Hon. Vice-Chancellor Dr. K. B. Kathiria and former Hon. Vice-Chancellor Dr. R. V. Vyas for their guidance and a keen interest in the timely progress of all project activities, in line with their expectations. Moreover, our Hon. Vice-Chancellor Dr. K. B. Kathiria has played a vital role in this prestigious project as the project was secured by the university when he was Director of Research & Dean P.G. studies. He is primarily responsible for all research projects, including national and international.

We are also thankful to Dr. (Ms) Anuradha Agrawal, National Coordinator (CAAST & Component 2) and Dr. Prabhat Kumar, Former National Coordinator, NAHEP- CAAST, ICAR, New Delhi, for their special interest in the implementation and growth of the project through their significant suggestions and the constant guidance in general and preparing this report in particular. We have also greatly benefitted from their office colleagues and staff, which is highly appreciable.

Helps rendered by the Director of Research & Dean P.G. Studies, Dr. M.K. Jhala, who is inter alia, responsible, in more ways than one, are thankfully acknowledged. His wholehearted support keen interest and professional way of monitoring of all activities pertaining to the project are highly encouraging and inspirational for all of us.

Dr. Y.C. Zala, Former Principal & Dean, International Agribusiness Management Institute and Officer In-charge has been deeply involved in all the activities since the inception of the project. The team thankfully acknowledges the assistance provided by Dr. Y.C. Zala.

We would like to acknowledge untiring efforts, leadership, and continuous guidance provided by Principal Investigator, NAHEP-CAAST, AAU which led to the completion and betterment of this book. We are also thankful for the collective efforts of whole team of NAHEP CAAST.

Place : Anand **Research Team**

Date : NAHEP-CAAST, AAU, Anand

Contents

Executive Summary

Poultry sector is one of the important sector of India. Poultry sector contributes Rs. 1347.57 billion in total output of livestock sector which hold 12.91 percent share in year 2019. The Indian poultry market was valued Rs. 2049 billion in 2019. The sector gives direct and indirect employment to 2.9 crore people in India. Poultry sector is presently emerging as sunrise sector with growth rate of 6-8 percent per annum. India is third largest producer of chicken egg and fifth largest producer of broilers/chicken meat in the world. The estimated production of egg production and meat production was 103.3 billion number and 4.06 million tonnes. The meat production from chicken has nearly fifty percent share in total meat production of country. Andhra Pradesh, Tamil Nadu and Telangana contribute more than 50 percent in total egg production. The model of contract broiler farming is adapted by majority of poultry farming for broiler. In broiler production Maharashtra, Haryana, West Bengal, Tamil Nadu and Andhra Pradesh are the leading producer. The annual per capita availability of egg was 79 eggs per annum. India's per capita consumption of broiler meat is 3.21 kg per person per year as compared to 58.5 kg in Israel, 49.8 kg in the United States, 46.7 kg in Malaysia and 43.9 kg in Australia. The unorganized sector (backyard poultry) supports the rural household with nutritional security, subsidiary income generation and provides the employment to women which increase the gender equality. India has twenty registered native chicken breeds. Different private and public sector has developed some dual-purpose breeds for backyard poultry like Grampriya, Gramshree, Kruilior etc. The egg production from deshi layer for the year 2018-19 is estimated to 2281.41 lakh numbers. In year 2018-19 the state contributes 1.79 percentages and holds fourteenth rank in India's egg production. Per capita availably of eggs is 28 eggs per annum for Gujarat state. Total chicken meat production from Gujarat in 2018-19 was 31131277 kg.

China is leading producer in egg production followed by European Union and United State of America. They hold share of about fifty percent in total egg production. Cal-Mine Foods of the United State of America has the highest number of layer birds (45 million). United states of America is the leading producer in chicken meat production with 19568042 tonnes production. JBS

S.A. of Brazil is the leading chicken meat producer with 4036 million head slaughtered annually.

Major poultry products which are traded in world market are live poultry, edible poultry meat, cuts & offals excluding livers, eggs in shells, eggs not in shell, egg yolks, egg powder etc. Brazil is the leading exporter of poultry products with export share of 19.12 percent in year 2018 followed by Netherland and United States of America. Germany is the major importer of poultry products in 2018 with share of 10.58 percent. India's share in world export is 0.21 percentages. Major market for Indian poultry products is Middle East and Asia. Some products like egg powder also exported to Japan and EU. Major exported poultry products are table eggs, egg powder, hatching eggs, SPF eggs, live birds, and poultry meat. Poultry products ranked 25th place in terms of total export with contribution of 637.3 Crore and share of 0.5 percent in India's export. Major importing countries of Indian poultry products are Oman, Maldives and Japan which hold share of According to the Sample Registration System baseline survey, 2014 released by the registrar general of India, 71 percentages of Indians over the age of 15 are non- vegetarian. India is a one of the major young population country in the world. So, there is a huge need to address the nutritional security of the people with higher protein diet. Thus, we have high requirement of protein to feed country's population in up-coming years and poultry products can become the cheapest source of nutrition.

The increase in per capita disposable income has led to an overall increase in food consumption, particularly protein in the form of meat and eggs. Preference of Indian consumer has changed and the cereals are now substituted with the animal products rather than a complementary product. The growth in the poultry with the growing demand and highly available supply because of integration with the organized sector, poultry products are more easily available and better price than other animal products. Consumers demand increase towards ready to eat/cook products. This leads to the market in more organized in urban sector with the spotlight on safety and hygiene standard and the more customer centric business models, supply chain remodeling and efficiencies driving value creation is expected in the sector.

Though, there is a huge potential in the poultry sector, it faces some challenges like regional imbalances in poultry production, underexploited poultry diversity, rising feed cost, emerging and re-emerging poultry diseases, poultry waste disposal and environmental concerns, climate change and associated stresses, lack of marketing infrastructure and seasonal demand.

1

Introduction

Indian poultry industry has made a fastest and remarkable growth ever since its inception and is presently emerging as a sunrise sector with a growth rate of 6-8 percent per annum. Today India is third largest producer of chicken egg and fifth largest producer of broilers/chicken meat in the world (Food and Agriculture Organization Corporate Statistical Database (FAOSTAT), 2018), with estimated production of 103.3 billion numbers eggs and 4.06 million tonnes of poultry meat in year 2018-19. Poultry sector contributes Rs.1347.57 billion in total output of livestock sector which hold 12.91 percent share (Basic Animal Husbandry Statistics (BAHS, 2019). The Indian poultry market was worth Rs.1,750 billion in 2018 and was worth Rs. 2,049 billion in 2019. The market is further projected to reach Rs. 4,340 billion by 2024, growing at a Compound Annual Growth Rate (CAGR) of 16.2 percent during 2019-2024 (www.indianmirror.com). The major growth drivers for the sector are increasing incomes coupled by changing food habits, large un-penetrated market, growth in the processing sector, and awareness of the consumer about the safe and hygienic poultry products. The sector has provided direct employment to 40 lakh and indirect employment to 2.5 crore people (Khan, 2019). The annual per capita availability of poultry products has increased from 5 eggs and 400 gram chicken in 1950 to 79 eggs and 3.21 kg chicken in 2019. However, it is far below then recommended consumption of 180 eggs and 10.8 kg poultry meat per person per annum by Indian Council of Medical Research.

The remarkable growth achieved in the Indian poultry sector is due to several factors like pure line breeding within the country in both public and private sectors leading to availability of elite commercial layer and broiler germplasm. The parallel development of other input sub-sectors like feed industry, hatcheries and farm appliances, poultry biological, vertical and horizontal integration in poultry farming and ever-increasing demand of poultry products have contributed to rapid growth.

The poultry sector in India has experienced a revolutionary shift in structure and operation, which has leads its transformation from a simple backyard activity to a major commercial agro based industry over a period of decades. The constant efforts in upgradation, modification and application of new technologies paved the way for the multifold and multifaceted growth in poultry and allied sectors. (Delgado *et al.,* 2003). In 2018-19 the share of the organized commercial sector and unorganized backyard farming is 82.2 and 18.8 respectively. Within the poultry sector, three fourth of the output (about 75.63%) is contributed by the broiler sector and other fourth (about 24.37%) by egg production. South India accounts for majority of total poultry production and consumption in the country. Andhra Pradesh, Tamil Nadu, Telangana, Karnataka and Kerala in south, Maharashtra in the west and Haryana and Punjab in the north are the key regions in poultry production.

In the poultry sector the development is not done only in production but also in productivity, sophistication and quality. India has developed high yielding layer (310- 340 eggs/year) and broiler (2.4-2.6 kg at 6 weeks) varieties together with standardized package of practices on nutrition, housing, management and disease control (Chatterjee and Rajkumar, 2015). This transformation has involved sizeable expansions and investments in breeding, hatching, rearing and processing. India is one of the few countries in the world that has put into place a sustained Specific Pathogen Free (SPF) egg production project. The poultry segment is mainly divided into three main segments including breeding, production and processing. Breeding segments includes the breeding and hatcheries industries; the production segment includes the commercial poultry farms, different integrators, poultry feed industries, equipment manufacturing industry and poultry healthcare industries; and the processing segment includes the different processing companies.

2

History of Poultry Sector

The word chicken originated from old English word 'icen', Germanic word 'kivkenam' and cock ('keuk'). According to Charles Darwin, the original chicken (Gallus domesticus) from which all modern domestic breeds of chicken have descended is referred to as Red Jungle Fowl (Gallus gallus). Archaeological discoveries in the Indus Valley suggest that chickens were probably domesticated from the Red Jungle fowl (Gallus gallus) as early as 5400 B.C. (West and Zhou, 1988). But there are some others who believe that modern chickens have been contributed by four wild species found in South East Asia. These were Gallus gallus (Red jungle fowl) found in eastern part of India, Burma, Java and Sumatra, Gallus sonneratii (Grey jungle fowl) prevalent in western and southern parts of India, Gallus lafayetti (Ceylone jungle fowl) the native of Sri Lanka and Gallus varius (Javan jungle fowl) found in lower adjacent islands of Java.

2.1. Origin of Modern Poultry

- 8000 BC

Archaeological evidence suggests that chicken existed in China

- 5400 BC

China - Cishan culture; but contribution of these birds to modern birds are doubtful.

- 3000 BC

In India account of cock fighting indicate that chicken have been part of the culture for a long time.

- 2500-2100 BC

Seals and toys bearing fowl images were excavated from Mohenjo-Daro. This suggested that the Harappa culture of Indus valley is the main source of diffusion of fowl through the world. Chicken used for sport.

- 1500 BC

Aryan migrated to India; included chicken in their culture but not as food.

- 1000-537 BC

Chicken had religious significance but forbidden as food; fighting cocks reached Persia.

- 200 BC

Chicken reached Egypt and got firmly established.

- 100 BC

Chicken reached Romans who knew about force- feeding, hybrid vigor, caponizing. Adopted chicken as food source and employed for cock fighting, religious purpose, superstition and divination.

- 1300 AD (Dawn of Christian era)

Chicken probably reached Europe and then to Russia. Due to fall of Roman Empire, importance of chicken in Europe reduced and become farmyard scavengers.

- 1500-1600 AD

Spanish conquest brought chickens to America and rapidly spread to South & Central America

2.2. Sequence of Domestication of Various Poultry Birds

Table 2.1: Sequence of domestication of various poultry birds

Species	Period	Country
Chicken	5400 BC	China – Cishan culture; but contribution of these birds to modern birds are doubtful
	2500 to 2100 BC	From Harappan culture of Indus valley; may be main source of diffusion through the world
Geese and Mallard ducks	2500 BC	China
	1500 BC	Egypt – separately domesticated ; in the west, mallard duck was not domesticated till middle age
Turkey	200 BC to 700 AD	Mexico
Japanese quail	11thCentury	Japan, China, Korea
Muscovy ducks	16th Century	Columbia, Peru
Guinea fowl	1500 AD	West African birds were introduced to Europe by Portuguese explorers

(*Source*: Sreenivasaiah, 2006)

2.3 Key Milestones in Indian Poultry Sector

Table 2.2: Key milestones in Indian poultry sector

Period		Achievement in Indian poultry sector
Pre-independence Scenario	•	Poultry considered as backyard activity with native birds such as Aseel, Kadaknath and other non-descriptive breeds without much attention to scientific practices and no concept of commercial farming observed.
	•	On recommendations of the Royal Commission on Agriculture in 1927, a poultry research section was established in 1939 at the Imperial Veterinary Research Institute, Izatnagar, which became a full-fledged poultry research division in 1952.
	•	Advanced training associateship of 2 years (on par with master's degree) was initiated in 1943 at Indian Council of Agricultural Research (ICAR) - Indian Veterinary Research Institute (IVRI).
	•	In the early 1940s, initial trials for vaccine against the dreaded Ranikhet Disease (RD) were started, which conferred immunity to birds and facilitated commercial farming.
I Five Year Plan (1951-56)	•	Commercial poultry keeping was promoted with launch of pilot project in Odisha.
	•	Breeds like White Leghorn (WLH), Rhode Island Red (RIR), and Black Minorca were considered for improving egg size and number.
	•	Selective breeding and proper development of poultry have also been included as a part of the key village scheme.
	•	ICAR-IVRI by a process of selective breeding has evolved an Indian strain (Hybrid WLH) which would substantially step up the yield.
	•	Effective vaccine against Ranikhet Disease (RD) was brought out.
	•	National diploma course in poultry production was initiated at ICAR-IVRI in 1952.
II Five Year Plan (1956-61)	•	The Central Poultry Breeding Farms laid the foundation for the development of poultry industry i.e., to acclimatize the genetically superior stock imported in 1956 from America under the Technical Cooperation Mission.
	•	Four multiplication farms with foreign collaboration were set up in the private sector for production of exotic chicks capable of laying 240 eggs a year.
	•	Up-gradation of indigenous germplasm through facilitated breeding with RIR and WLH.
	•	Problems of cold storage facilities and other diseases were recognized.

Period		**Achievement in Indian poultry sector**
	•	Poultry science department started in Acharya N. G. Ranga Agricultural University, Hyderabad and Punjab Agricultural University, Ludhiana (1960).
	•	Duck development programmes have been initiated on a small scale during early 1960's.
III Five Year Plan (1961-66)	•	Poultry stocks are imported from Australia (1965) for government breeding farms under 'Freedom from Hunger Campaign'.
	•	Intensive Poultry Development Projects (IPDP) were announced for promoting profitable poultry keeping.
	•	Expansion and strengthening of infrastructure of state & regional poultry farms and extension-cum-development centers.
	•	Meat type strains were imported from Israel.
IV Five Year Plan (1969-74)	•	Growth of ancillary industries like poultry feed, equipment and sales organisations for egg and meat was promoted.
	•	Propagation of stock with high Feed Conversion Ratio (FCR).
	•	Proposed to take up a coordinated poultry breeding programme at central and state farms to evolve superior lines and exploit hybrid vigour. This is the foundation for All India Coordinated Research Project (AICRP) on poultry breeding (1970).
	•	Establishment of poultry science division at Chennai, Mannuthy, Hisar and Bangalore.
	•	Launching of centre of excellence with a support from United Nations Development Programme (UNDP) at poultry science division, ICAR-IVRI (1972).
	•	Random Sample Poultry Performance Test (RSPPT) centre was established at Hessarghatta (1970) for layer and broiler varieties of genetic stock.
	•	Central poultry training institute was established in 1972.
V Five Year Plan (1974-79)	•	Particular emphasis has been laid on scientific poultry breeding programme.
	•	Cage rearing of layers was initiated.
	•	Country started importing Cobb strain.
	•	Poultry Science division was initiated at Bombay and Bhubaneswar.
	•	ICAR- Central Avian Research Institute (CARI)emerged from Poultry Science division in ICAR-IVRI. Central duck breeding farm was established to introduce high yielding duck varieties under Ministry of Agriculture, Government of India in 1981 with technical collaboration of United Kingdom.

Period		Achievement in Indian poultry sector
VI Five Year Plan (1980-85)	•	An aggressive consumer education programme became major component of market promotion activity.
	•	National Agricultural Cooperative Marketing Federation of India Ltd (NAFED) interference in poultry eggs and meat marketing at national and export level.
	•	Market surveys in the country and abroad taken place from time to time.
	•	National Egg Coordination Committee (NECC) established in the country.
	•	Banking sectors started supporting poultry production.
	•	Emergence of feed and pharmaceutical industries.
	•	Entry of private sectors in poultry production.
	•	Broiler farming (not in integrated but isolated form) became popular.
	•	Propagation of pure line broiler stock.
	•	Multiple batch farms in urban areas started operating.
	•	Poultry Science education started at Akola and Namakkal veterinary colleges.
	•	Centre for advanced studies in poultry science was established at Mannuthy, Kerala.
VII Five Year Plan (1985-90)	•	At the Central Poultry Breeding Farms, poultry strains like HH260 and BH-78 were evolved released to commercial farms.
	•	ICAR developed high egg-laying strains like ILI-80 and fast growing broiler strains such as IBL-80 and 18B-for release.
	•	111 egg and poultry production-cum-marketing centers were established during the plan period.
	•	A National Hatchery Registration Programme was also introduced during the plan period to enforce production and supply of quality chicks of both layer and broiler types.
	•	Dr. B.V. Rao Institute of Poultry Management and Technology was established at Pune, Maharashtra (1987).
	•	Directorate of Poultry Research at Hyderabad was established to co-ordinate the AICRP activities across the country.
VIII Five Year Plan (1992-97)	•	High yield layers/broilers have been developed and private entrepreneurship was encouraged.
	•	Poultry production by private units and co-operatives was promoted. Subsequently concerned organizations were encouraged by providing suitable inputs like finance, appropriate training and guidance.
	•	Quail, duck and guinea fowl rearing farms were established at state poultry centers.

Period		Achievement in Indian poultry sector
	•	Scientific turkey farms with imported stocks of Broad Breasted Large, White and Bronze (pure lines) was initiated in 1995.
	•	Additional cold storage facilities for storing eggs and meat at selected districts have been created to overcome variation in production and demand.
	•	India's first egg processing plant established at Hyderabad with annual capacity of 3,000 tonnes egg powder.
	•	High raised platform cages, vertical integration, corporate tendency in layer production took a boost.
	•	Contract farming system introduced in broiler production.
	•	All in all out batch system concept led the broiler industry.
	•	Marketing risk for farmer excluded.
	•	Rural based production promoted.
	•	Improvement of biosecurity measures.
	•	Import of grandparent stocks was commenced.
IX Five Year Plan (1997-02)	•	Poultry sub-sector has also made significant progress due to research and development activities. The egg production which was at the level of 22 billion nos. during1991-92 increased to 28.2 billion during 1996-97. The per-capita availability of eggs increased from 25 to 30 per annum, for the same period.
	•	Establishment of a pyramid-programme for low-input technology bird dissemination and stock propagation through ICAR, State universities, Government of India (GoI) organisations and subsequent by multiplication of Grand Parents /parent stock in CPDO. Multiplication of parents into commercial stock through strengthening of infrastructure of state farms.
	•	'Gramapriya' the taker of rural poultry breed developed and released at 46th livestock and poultry show.
	•	Robotics intervention in commercial poultry housing, feeding, egg collection, manure disposal, poultry processing and value addition.
	•	Poultry housing scenario has been changed with the advent of environmentally controlled housing models.
	•	Capacity achieved to enter into export market.
	•	Establishment of egg production plants.
	•	Growth of integrators; mammoth hatcheries and feed mills.
	•	Inclusion of growth promoters in broiler and layer feeding.
X Five Year Plan (2002-07)	•	Strategies for commercial broiler and layer production have been established and become successful.
	•	Poultry products export has been given importance.

Period		Achievement in Indian poultry sector
	•	Steps for the development of infrastructure like cold-storage, pressured air cargo capacity and reference laboratory for the certification of health and products.
	•	Central Poultry Development Organisation (CPDO) was emerged at North, East, West and Southern regions.
XI Five Year Plan (2007- 12)	•	Government emphasized on rural poultry development through centrally sponsored schemes.
	•	Poultry estates, poultry development and poultry venture capital fund scheme were launched to implement private participation and entrepreneurship development to achieve sustainable poultry production.
	•	Rural Backyard Poultry Development Project was launched in 2009
	•	ICAR Initiated poultry seed project mainly to popularize rural poultry production with superior germplasm (Vanaraja and Gramapriya).
	•	High capacity farms operating with low margin.
	•	Entry of broiler breeding giants.
	•	Growth performance of poultry under Indian conditions matching world standards.
XII Five Year Plan (2012-2017)	•	Rural poultry component is included in AICRP to develop location specific germplasm for rural poultry.
	•	Institutionalization of contract broiler farming.

3

Poultry Sector Scenario

Poultry sector has been divided into two broad classes based on the management practices. First one is commercial poultry farming which is the well-organized sector. Second one is backyard poultry farming which plays supportive role for rural economy. The commercial farming practices can divide into two subclasses: layer and broiler industry. Commercial poultry farming provides primary source of income to the farmers and widely influenced by market driven forces. Backyard poultry farming comprises dual purpose birds as both layer and broiler. It supports the rural household with nutritional security, subsidiary income generation and provides the employment to women which

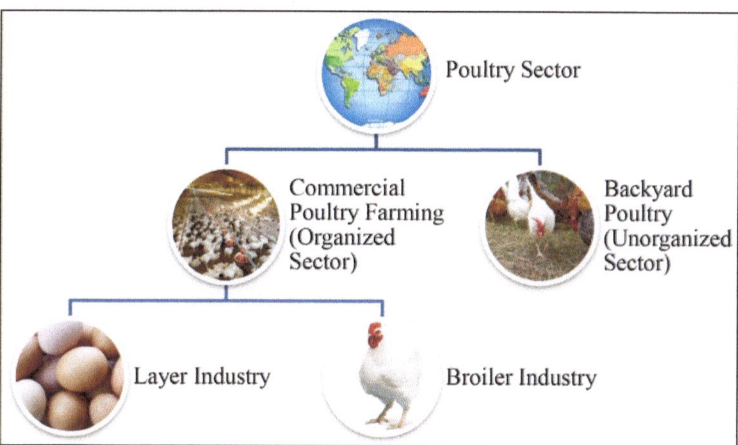

Fig. 3.1: Scenario of poultry sector

Egg production by backyard and commercial poultry farm

Out of total egg production of 103.3 billion numbers eggs, commercial poultry farming is producing 84.91 billion number eggs whereas, backyard poultry farming is producing 18.41 billion numbers contributing 82.2 percent and 17.8 percent of total production of egg respectively (BAHS, 2019).

4

Commercial Poultry Farming (Organized Sector)

4.1 Layer Industry

4.1.1 Global scenario

Poultry is raised by approximately 80 percent of rural households in developing countries. Food and Agriculture Organization's statistics department show that total egg production has grown from 61.7 million tonnes in 2008 to 76.7 million tonnes in 2018. China continues to lead the way, producing 466 billion eggs in 2018, which represents 34 percent of the global market. China has been the world's largest producer of eggs for the last 30 years. China, European Union (EU), United states of America (USA) and India produce almost 60 percent of the world's eggs, while the next 6 largest producers take a further 16 percent of the market. This means that the top 10 egg producers account for more than three fourth of the world's egg production. Asia is the largest egg-producing region, with more than 60 percent of global output.

Table 4.1: Top ten egg producers in the world

Sr. No.	Country	Production (Billion Number)	Share of world market (%)
1	China	466	34
2	EU	120	9
3	United states of America	109	8
4	India	95	7
5	Mexico	57	4
6	Brazil	53	4
7	Russion Federation	44	3
8	Japan	44	3
9	Indonesia	38	3
10	Turkey	20	1

(Source: FAOSTAT, 2018)

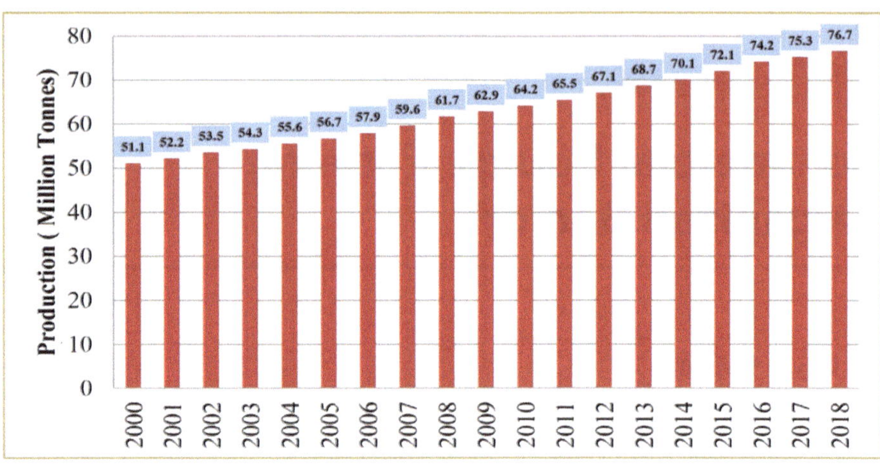

Fig. 4.1: Development of global egg production, 2000 – 2018 (FAOSTAT, 2018)

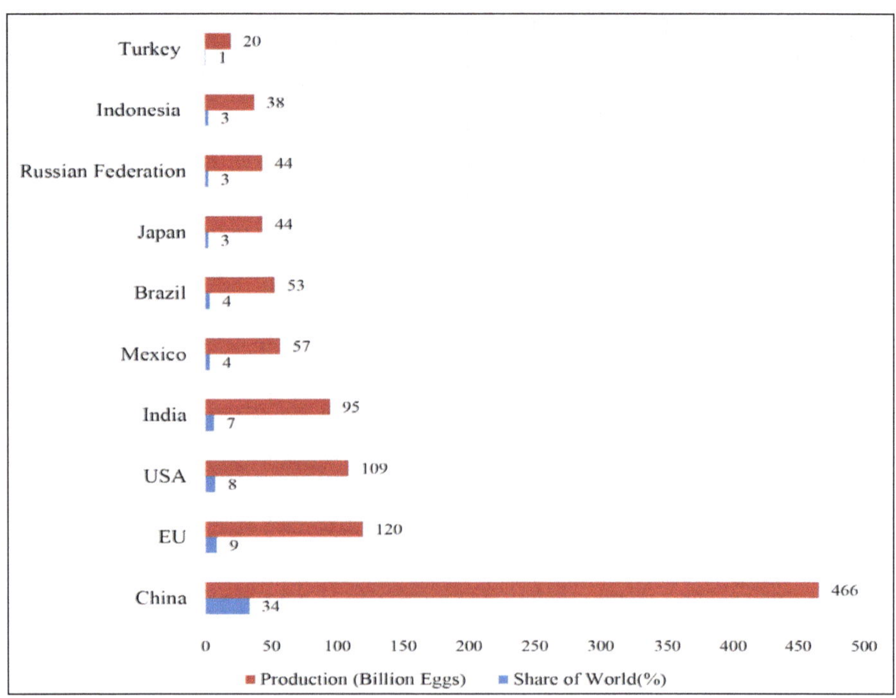

Fig. 4.2: Top ten egg producing countries (FAOSTAT, 2018)

The ranking of the top companies in terms of number layers is indicated in table 4.2.

Table 4.2: Top companies in the world in terms of number of layers

Rank	Company	Country	Layers (in million)
1	Cal-Maine Foods	United States	45.0
2	Proteína Animal (PROAN)	Mexico	34.0
3	Rose Acre Farms	United States	26.6
4	CP Group	Thailand	22.0
5	Versova Holdings LLC	United States	21.0
6	Hillandale Farms	United States	20.0
7	Ise Inc.	Japan	20.0
8	Arab Company for Livestock Development (ACOLID)	Saudi Arabia	14.4
9	Daybreak Foods	United States	14.0
10	Michael Foods	United States	13.3
11	Kazi Farms Group	Bangladesh	12.7
12	Industrias Bachoco	Mexico	12.2
13	Empresas Guadalupe	Mexico	12.0
14	Rembrandt Enterprises	United States	11.9
15	CP Standart Gida Sanayi Ve Ticaret (CP Turkey)	Turkey	11.0
16	MPS Egg Farms	United States	10.9
17	Center Fresh Group	United States	10.8
18	Prairie Star Farms	United States	10.8
19	Avangardco	Ukraine	10.5
20	Granja Mantiqueira	Brazil	10.5

(*Source*: Clements, 2020)

4.1.2 Indian Scenario

The total egg production in the country was 1.832 billion nos. in the year 1950-51 and since production of the eggs increase over a period of time, as depicted in the table below. There has been remarkable growth in production of eggs up to the year 1999-2000. From the year 1999-2000 onwards the production of egg improved substantially and it reached 103.32 billion nos. in 2018-19. The per capita availability was 5 eggs per annum during the period 1950-51. There has been steady increase in per capita availability of egg since then till 2018-19 with marginal fluctuations in the intermittent periods. The per capita availability reached at 79 eggs per annum in the year 2018-19 from 74 eggs per annum from previous year 2017-18.

Table 4.3: Egg production and per capita availability of egg

Years	Eggs production (in Billion Nos.)	Human population (in Crore)	Per capita availability (in No./Annum)
1950-1951	1.83	35.9	5
1955-1956	1.91	39.3	5
1960-1961	2.88	43.4	7
1968-1969	5.30	51.8	10
1973-1974	7.76	58.0	13
1979-1980	9.52	66.4	14
1980-1981	10.06	67.9	15
1981-1982	10.88	69.2	16
1982-1983	11.45	70.8	16
1983-1984	12.79	72.3	18
1984-1985	14.25	73.9	19
1985-1986	16.13	75.5	21
1986-1987	17.31	77.1	22
1987-1988	17.80	78.8	23
1988-1989	18.98	80.5	24
1989-1990	20.20	82.2	25
1990-1991	21.10	83.9	25
1991-1992	21.98	85.6	26
1992-1993	22.93	87.2	26
1993-1994	24.17	89.2	27
1994-1995	25.98	91.0	29
1995-1996	27.20	92.8	29
1996-1997	27.50	94.6	29
1997-1998	28.69	96.4	30
1998-1999	29.48	98.3	30
1999-2000	30.45	100.1	30
2000-2001	36.63	101.9	36
2001-2002	38.73	104.0	37
2002-2003	39.82	105.6	38
2003-2004	40.40	107.2	38
2004-2005	45.20	108.9	42
2005-2006	46.24	110.6	42
2006-2007	50.66	112.2	45
2007-2008	53.58	113.8	47
2008-2009	55.56	115.4	48
2009-2010	60.27	117.0	52
2010-2011	63.02	118.6	53
2011-2012	66.45	121.0	55
2012-2013	69.73	121.2	58

Years	Eggs production (in Billion Nos.)	Human population (in Crore)	Per capita availability (in No./Annum)
2013-2014	74.75	122.8	61
2014-2015	78.48	124.4	63
2015-2016	82.93	126.0	66
2016-2017	88.14	127.5	69
2017-2018	95.22	129.0	74
2018-2019	103.32	130.5	79

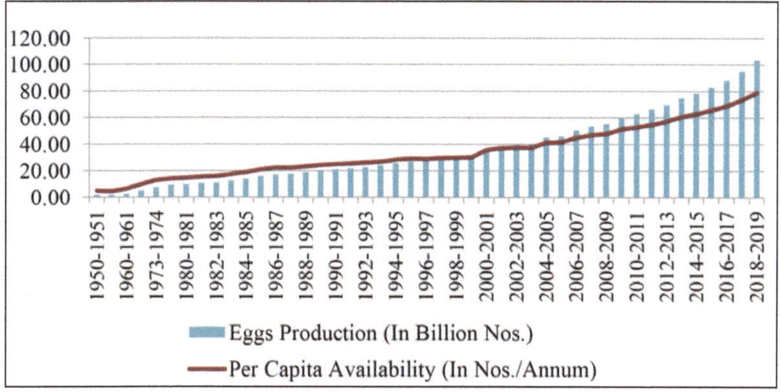

Fig. 4.3: Egg production and per capita availability of egg

Annual Growth Rate of Egg Production of Last Ten Years

Figure 4.4 shows the annual growth rate of egg production during the period 200910 to 2018-19. As compared to 2017-18, the growth rate of the current year 2018-19 also shows a significant improvement in the egg production with the growth registered as 8.51 percent. It is seen that the annual growth rate has crossed over 8 percent during the last two reference period.

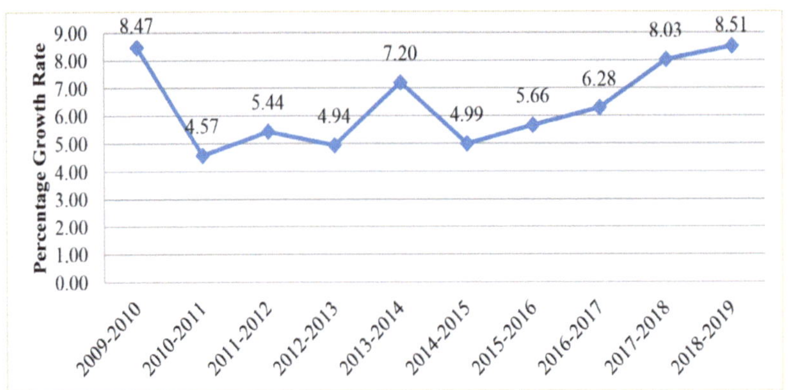

Fig. 4.4: Annual growth rate of egg production

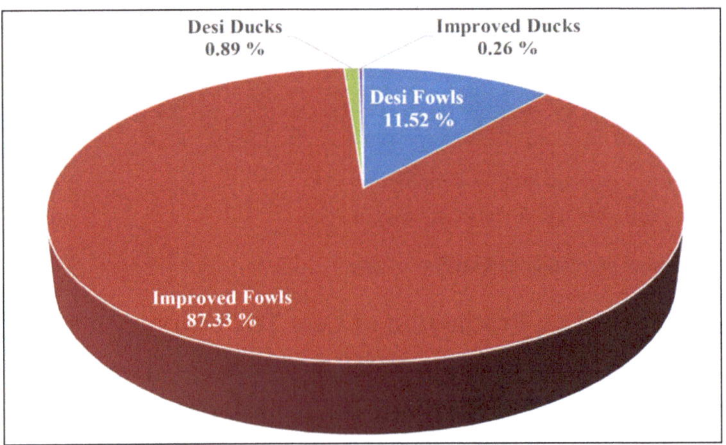

Fig. 4.5: Species-wise share of egg production in 2018-19

Figure 4.5 depicts the contribution of egg production by Fowl and Duck. The graph shows Improved Fowl contribute 87.33 percent of the production of egg and 11.52 percent is from Desi Fowls with respect to total production of egg. The Desi Duck and Improved Duck contribute 0.89 percent and 0.26 percent, respectively with respect to total egg production.

Overall trends in layer industry

Table 4.4: Trends in layer industry

Sr.No	Parameter	1990	2015
1	Layer birds (crore)	10	24
2	Layer feed price (Rs)	12	22
3	Egg price (Rs)	1.5	2.90
4	Eggs per head/ year	20	68

5	Eggs per hen	260	310
6	Average layer farm size	20000	200000
7	Separate brooding (%)	10	80
8	Feed automation (%)	10	80
9	Eggs cleaning and packing	No	Important

(*Source*: Kotaiah, 2016)

Table 4.5: Genetic progress in White and Brown egg layers

Traits	**White Layer**		**Brown Layer**	
Year	2000	2020	2000	2020
2020 Egg numbers hen housed (at 75 weeks)	324	364	319	361
Egg numbers hen housed (at 90 weeks)		444		440
Egg numbers hen housed (at 100 weeks)		505		495
Maximum lay rate (%)	95	97	95	97
Egg mass (kg. at 75 weeks)	20,5	22,7	20,0	22,6
Egg mass (kg. at 90 weeks)		28		27,7
Egg mass (kg. at 100 weeks)		32		31,4
Daily feed intake (grams)	110	109	114	112
Feed conversion (grams feed/grams egg mass)	2,18	1,98	2,31	2,07
Liveability (% at 90 weeks)	94	95	93	94

State wise scenario of India

Statewise egg production is shown in the table 4.5. which shows that, during 2014-15 to 2018-19, there is a steady increase in the production in all states except for the states like Kerala where the trend in the production estimates somewhat fluctuates.

Table 4.6 : Egg production during 2014-15 to 2018-19 of different States (Figures in billion Number) (Source: BAHS, 2019)

Sr.No	**States/ UT**	**2014-15**	**2015-16**	**2016-17**	**2017-18**	**2018-19**
1	Andhra Pradesh	13.10	14.17	15.83	17.78	19.75
2	Tamil Nadu	15.93	16.13	16.68	17.42	18.84
3	Telangana	10.62	11.21	11.82	12.67	13.69
4	West Bengal	4.81	6.01	6.55	7.64	8.60
5	Haryana	4.58	4.91	5.21	5.59	6.06
6	Karnataka	4.40	4.77	5.07	5.57	6.00
7	Maharashtra	5.08	5.29	5.48	5.70	5.96
8	Punjab	4.26	4.42	4.78	5.23	5.59
9	Uttar Pradesh	2.08	2.19	2.29	2.44	2.61
10	Odisha	1.92	1.93	1.97	2.06	2.35
11	Kerala	2.50	2.44	2.34	2.35	2.29
12	Madhya Pradesh	1.18	1.44	1.69	1.94	2.14
13	Chhattisgarh	1.47	1.50	1.66	1.77	1.89

Sr.No	States/ UT	2014-15	2015-16	2016-17	2017-18	2018-19
14	Gujarat	1.66	1.72	1.79	1.79	1.85
15	Rajasthan	1.32	1.39	1.36	1.45	1.66
16	Bihar	0.98	1.00	1.11	1.22	1.28
17	Jharkhand	0.47	0.48	0.51	0.55	0.64
18	Assam	0.47	0.47	0.48	0.50	0.50
19	Uttarakhand	0.37	0.39	0.41	0.43	0.45
20	Tripura	0.20	0.22	0.23	0.26	0.28
21	Jammu & Kashmir	0.50	0.23	0.23	0.23	0.23
22	A&N Islands	0.09	0.10	0.10	0.11	0.11
23	Meghalaya	0.11	0.11	0.11	0.11	0.11
24	Manipur	0.11	0.10	0.10	0.10	0.11
25	Himachal Pradesh	0.11	0.08	0.10	0.10	0.10
26	Arunachal Pradesh	0.04	0.04	0.05	0.06	0.06
27	Mizoram	0.04	0.04	0.04	0.04	0.04
28	Nagaland	0.04	0.05	0.04	0.04	0.04
29	Goa	0.01	0.04	0.03	0.03	0.03
30	Chandigarh	0.02	0.02	0.02	0.02	0.02
31	Lakshadweep	0.01	0.01	0.01	0.01	0.01
32	Puducherry	0.01	0.01	0.01	0.01	0.01
33	Sikkim	0.01	0.01	0.01	0.01	0.01
34	Daman & Diu	0.00	0.00	0.00	0.00	0.00
35	D.& N. Haveli	0.01	0.01	0.01	0.01	0.00
36	Delhi	0.00	0.00	0.00	0.00	0.00
	All India	78.48	82.93	88.14	95.22	103.32

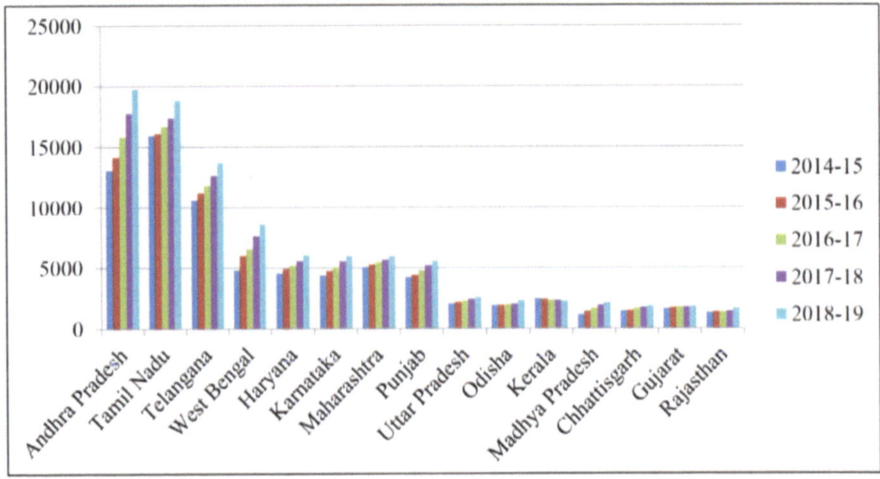

Fig. 4.6: Egg production of major egg producing states

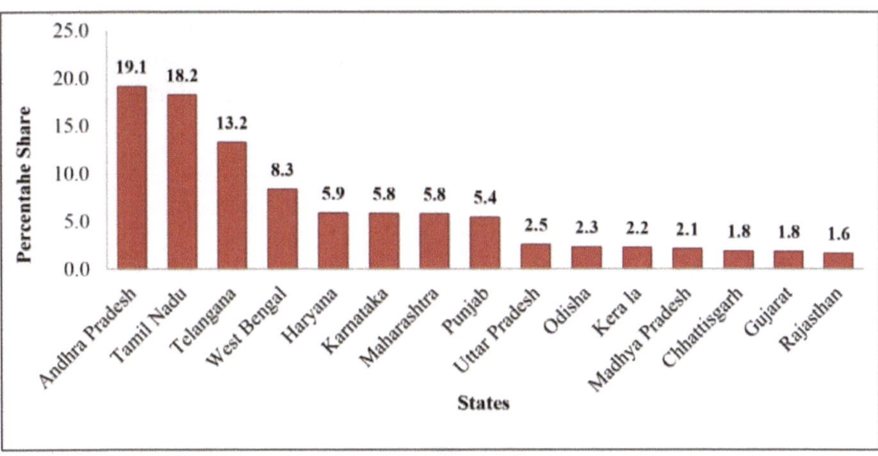

Fig. 4.7: Percentage share of egg production of major egg producing states

The largest producer of egg is Andhra Pradesh which produces 19.1 percent of the total egg production in the country followed by Tamil Nadu that produces 18.2 percent of the total egg production. Telangana is the third largest egg producing state in the country with a share of 13.2 percent of the total egg production in the country. Some other States that contribute more than 5 percent in the total egg produced across country are West Bengal, Haryana, Karnataka, Maharashtra and Punjab. All together only three states i.e. Andhra Pradesh, Tamil Nadu and Telangana contributes around 50 percent of total egg production.

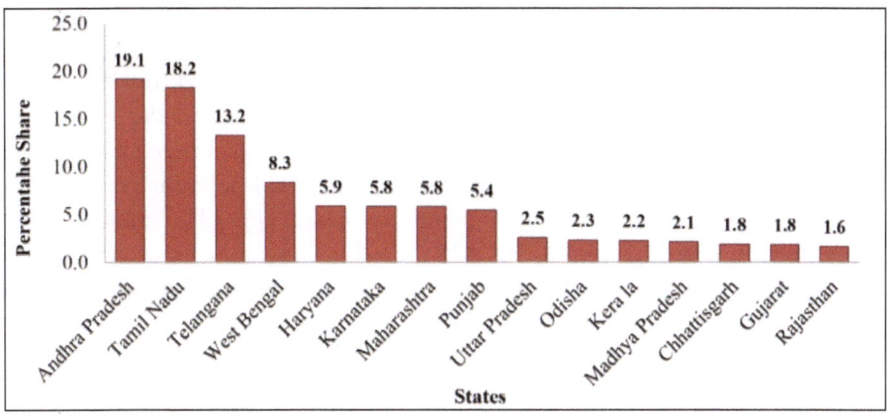

Fig. 4.8: Annual growth rate of egg production of fifteen major egg producing state/UTs

The state-wise analysis in the growth pattern of egg production during 2018-19 has shown in figure. 4.8. Five states viz. Rajasthan, Odisha, West Bengal,

Andhra Pradesh and Madhya Pradesh have crossed the national growth rate and registered the significant growth in egg production. The graph also denotes that 9 States/UTs have registered growth above 7.5 percent during 2018-19 in case of Egg production.

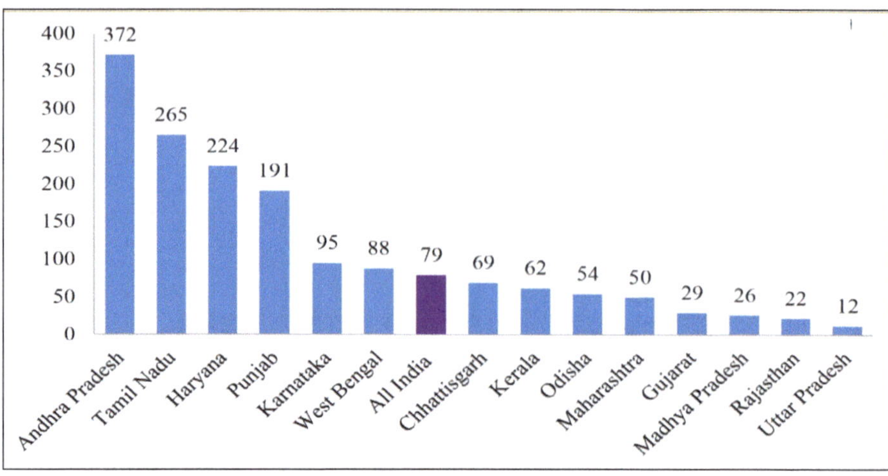

Fig. 4.9: Per capita availability of eggs for the year 2018-19 of major egg producing states

Figure 4.9 shows the per-capita availability of egg during 2018-19 in various states/ UTs including the all India average. 6 States are having per-capita availability more than the national average.

4.1.3. Gujarat State Scenario

The estimated population of deshi layer during the year 2018-19 is 15403 hundred, which shows an increase of 0.03 percent compared to the previous year. The estimated population of total dashy poultry works out during the year 2018-19 is 45347 hundred, which shows a decrease of 1.73 percent compared to the previous year. The estimated average egg yield per year per layer for dashi poultry for the year 2018-19 comes to 148.12 eggs. The corresponding figure for the year 2017-2018 was 145.28 eggs. Thus, this shows an increase of 1.95 percent in productivity of deshi layer for the year 2017-18 as compared to the previous year.

Table 4.7: Details of poultry production in Gujarat state

Sr.No.	Items	Unit	2017-18 ('00)	2018-19 ('00)	% of Increase or decrease over previous year
1	**Layers Poultry Population**				
	Deshi	00 No.	15398	15403	0.03
	Improved	00 No.	51839	54047	4.26
	Total	00 No.	67237	69450	3.29
	Total poultry				
	Deshi	00 No.	46143	45347	-1.73
	Improved	00 No.	64503	65404	1.4
	Total	00 No.	110647	110750	0.09
2	**Yield per layer per year**				
	Deshi	No.	145.28	148.12	1.95
	Improved	No.	301.52	300.89	-0.21
3	**Production**				
	Deshi	Lakh No.	2237.05	2281.41	1.98
	Improved	Lakh No.	15630.66	16262.4	4.04
	Total	Lakh No.	17867.71	18543.8	3.78

(Source: Directorate of Animal Husbandry (DOAH), 2020)

The egg production from deshi layer for the year 2018-19 is estimated to 2281.41 lakh numbers as compared to 2237.06 lakh numbers estimated for the year 2017-18 showing an increase of 1.98 percent over the previous year.

The estimated population of improved layer and improved total poultry works out during the year under report is 54047 hundred and 65404 hundred respectively, showing an increase of 4.26 percent and 1.40 percent over previous year respectively.

Table 4.8 shows the egg production of Gujarat and share of its contribution in total production for the year 2008-09 to 2018-2019. In year 2018-19 the state contributes 1.79 percentages and holds the rank of fourteen.

Table 4.8: The estimates of egg production of Gujarat comparison with India

Sr.No.	Year	Gujarat (Lakh Nos.)	India (Lakh Nos.)	% Contribution	Rank
1	2008-09	12675.00	555624.00	2.28	10
2	2009-10	12762.00	602671.00	2.12	10
3	2010-11	13269.00	630244.00	2.11	10
4	2011-12	14269.00	664499.00	2.15	11
5	2012-13	14558.40	697307.00	2.09	11
6	2013-14	15550.74	747518.80	2.08	10
7	2014-15	16565.00	784839.00	2.11	12
8	2015-16	17216.00	829294.00	2.08	12

Sr.No.	Year	Gujarat (Lakh Nos.)	India (Lakh Nos.)	% Contribution	Rank
9	2016-17	17940.00	881372.00	2.04	12
10	2017-18	17868.00	952173.00	1.88	13
11	2018-19	18544.00	1033176.00	1.79	14

(Source: DOAH, 2020)

Total egg production for the year 2018-19 was 18544 lakh which is 3.78 percent higher than previous year. Per capita availability of egg was 28 eggs/ annum.

Table 4.9: Year wise egg production and per capita availability of egg

Year	Deshi (Lakh No)	% change over previous year	Improved (Lakh No)	% change over previous year	Total (Lakh No)	% change over previous year	Per capita availability (No /Year)
1994-95	1287		3395		4682		
1995-96	1292	0.39	3650	7.51	4942	5.55	
1996-97	1367	5.80	3650	0	5017	1.52	
1997-98	1384	1.24	3501	-4.08	4885	-2.63	
1998-99	1448	4.59	3224	-7.92	4671	-4.38	
1999-00	1465	1.24	3306	2.55	4771	2.14	
2000-01	1457	-0.58	2003	-39.41	3460	-27.48	7
2001-02	1277	-12.35	2424	21.02	3701	6.97	7
2002-03	1247	-2.35	2601	7.30	3848	3.97	7
2003-04	1159	-7.06	3265	25.53	4423	14.94	8
2004-05	1223	5.52	3808	16.63	5031	13.75	9
2005-06	1296	5.97	4479	17.62	5775	14.79	11
2006-07	1447	11.65	6311	40.90	7757	34.32	14
2007-08	1497	3.46	6760	7.11	8256	6.43	15
2008-09	1485	-0.80	11191	65.55	12675	53.52	22
2009-10	1526	2.76	11236	0.40	12762	0.69	22
2010-11	1635	7.17	11634	3.54	13269	3.98	23
2011-12	1745	6.70	12524	7.65	14269	7.54	23
2012-13	1791	2.65	12767	1.94	14558	2.03	23
2013-14	1810	1.07	13740	7.62	15550	6.81	24
2014-15	2078	14.79	14487	5.43	16565	6.53	25
2015-16	2412	16.05	14804	2.19	17216	3.93	26
2016-17	2274	-5.73	15667	5.83	17940	4.21	27
2017-18	2237	-1.61	15631	-0.23	17868	-0.40	27
2018-19	2281	1.98	16262	4.04	18544	3.78	28

(*Source*: DOAH, 2020)

Average annual growth rate in different financial year was higher in the fifth Five Year Plan (FYP). It was 4.70 percentage for the FYP of 2012-13 to 2016-17.

Table 4.10: Average annual growth rate (%) as per FYP in egg production

Five Year Plan	Growth Rate (%) in Egg Production
1980-81 to 1984-85	5.54
1985-86 to 1989-90	8.83
1992-93 to 1996-97	1.92
1997-98 to 2001-02	-5.08
2002-03 to 2006-07	16.35
2007-08 to 2011-12	14.43
2012-13 to 2016-17	4.70

(*Source*: DOAH, 2020)

Annual growth rate for the current decade (2010-11 to 2018-19) is 4.43 percent.

Table 4.11: Annual growth rates as per decadal year

Year	Growth rate (%) in egg production
1980-81 to 1990-91	7.14
1990-91 to 2000-01	-1.14
2000-01 to 2010-11	15.34
2010-11 to 2018-19	4.43

(*Source*: DOAH, 2020)

Table 4.12: Category and district-wise egg production in Gujarat State (2018-19) (Production in lakh nos.) (Source: DOAH, 2020)

Deshi Layer				Improved Layer				Total Egg Production			
Rank	**Name of the District**	**Desi Layer**	**Share (%)**	**Rank**	**Name of the District**	**Improved Layer**	**Share (%)**	**Rank**	**Name of the District**	**Total Layer**	**Share (%)**
1	Valsad	389.31	17.06	1	Anand	8504.66	52.30	1	Anand	8513.20	45.91
2	Panchmahals	270.03	11.84	2	Bhavnagar	2791.69	17.17	2	Bhavnagar	2803.15	15.12
3	Surat	240.84	10.56	3	Alunedabad	1393.74	8.57	3	Alunedabad	1403.41	7.57
4	Tapi	236.30	10.36	4	Surat	630.87	3.88	4	Surat	871.72	4.70
5	Vadodara	215.32	9.44	5	Navsari	576.31	3.54	5	Navsari	765.58	4.13
6	Dahod	194.19	8.51	6	Kheda	513.13	3.16	6	Valsad	712.21	3.84
7	Navsari	189.27	8.30	7	Valsad	322.90	1.99	7	Kheda	537.25	2.90
8	Bharuch	125.70	5.51	8	Rajkot	269.04	1.65	8	Tapi	461.98	2.49
9	Dang	101.31	4.44	9	Tapi	225.68	1.39	9	Vadodara	407.46	2.20
10	Narmada	88.44	3.88	10	Vadodara	192.14	1.18	10	Rajkot	273.97	1.48
11	Sabarkantha	56.08	2.46	11	Jamnagar	178.51	1.10	11	Panchmahals	270.03	1.46
12	Banaskantha	37.67	1.65	12	Patan	144.48	0.89	12	Dahod	194.19	1.05
13	Junagadh	31.34	1.37	13	Junagadh	121.96	0.75	13	Jamnagar	185.93	1.00
14	Kheda	24.12	1.06	14	Banaskantha	119.87	0.74	14	Bharuch	174.22	0.94
15	Patan	12.89	0.57	15	Mahesana	96.72	0.59	15	Banaskantha	157.53	0.85
16	Bhavnagar	11.45	0.50	16	Porbandar	75.57	0.46	16	Patan	157.37	0.85
17	Alunedabad	9.67	0.42	17	Bharuch	48.52	0.30	17	Junagadh	153.3	0.83
18	Anand	8.54	0.37	18	Sabarkantha	45.43	0.28	18	Mahesana	104.37	0.56
19	Mahesana	7.66	0.34	19	Gandhinagar	11.16	0.07	19	Sabarkantha	101.51	0.55
20	Jamnagar	7.42	0.33	20	Surendranagar	0	0.00	20	Dang	101.31	0.55
21	Kachchh	7.17	0.31	21	Panchmahals	0	0.00	21	Narmada	88.44	0.48
22	Amreli	5.75	0.25	22	Narmada	0	0.00	22	Porbandar	76.34	0.41

Deshi Layer				Improved Layer				Total Egg Production			
Rank	**Name of the District**	**Desi Layer**	**Share (%)**	**Rank**	**Name of the District**	**Improved Layer**	**Share (%)**	**Rank**	**Name of the District**	**Total Layer**	**Share (%)**
23	Rajkot	4.92	0.22	23	Kachchh	0	0.00	23	Gandhinagar	15.18	0.08
24	Gandhinagar	4.01	0.18	24	Dang	0	0.00	24	Kachchh	7.17	0.04
25	Surendranagar	1.23	0.05	25	Dahod	0	0.00	25	Amreli	5.75	0.03
26	Porbandar	0.78	0.03	26	Amreli	0	0.00	26	Surendranagar	1.23	0.01
Gujarat State		**2281.41**	**100.00**	**Gujarat State**		**16262.4**	**100.00**	**Gujarat State**		**18543.8**	**100.00**

4.2 Broiler Industry

4.2.1 Global Scenario

Poultry meat represented about 37 percent of global meat production. The United States of America is the world's largest poultry meat producer, with 18 percent of global output, followed by China, Brazil and the Russian Federation. To meet growing demand, world poultry meat production soared from 9 to 128.8 million tonnes between 1961 and 2018. India ranked 5th in world chicken meat production in the world in 2018 (FAOSTAT, 2018).

Table 4.13: Major chicken meat producer in the world in 2018

Rank	Country	Production (Tonnes)
1	United States of America	19568042
2	Brazil	14914563
3	China	14578673
4	Russian Federation	4543002
5	India	3590525

(Source: FAOSTAT, 2018)

Table 4.14: Top ten poultry meat consuming countries (Total consumption)

Sr.No	Country	Consumption ('000 Tonnes)
1	China	19,028
2	United States	18,044
3	European Union	14,013
4	Brazil	8,893
5	Russia	5,159
6	Mexico	4,072
7	India	3,257
8	Japan	2,444
9	South Africa	2,312
10	Iran	2,114

(Source: OECD FAO Agricultural Outlook 2018-2027)

Table 4.15: Top ten poultry meat consumers (Per capita consumption)

Sr. No	Country	kg per capita
1	Israel	58.5
2	United State	49.8
3	Malaysia	46.7
4	Australia	43.9
5	Brazil	40.6
6	Argentina	40.4
7	Saudi Arabia	40.0
8	New Zealand	37.4
9	Chile	36.1
10	South Africa	36.1

(Source: OECD FAO Agricultural Outlook 2018-2027, 2018 estimates.)

India's per capita consumption of broiler meat is 3.21 kg per person per year as compared to 58.5 kg in Israel, 49.8 kg in the United States, 46.7kg in Malaysia, 43.9 kg in Australia, and 17 kg for the world. Consumption of broiler meat is increasing at a faster pace in developing nations, like Brazil, Argentina and Chile.

Table 4.16: Leading chicken meat producer in the world

Rank	Company	Country	No of head slaughtered annually (in millions)
1	JBS S.A.	Brazil	4036.0
2	Tyson Foods	United States	1991.6
3	BRF	Brazil	1554.0
4	New Hope Liuhe	China	1300.0
5	Wen's Food Group	China	748.0
6	CP Group	Thailand	685.0
7	Koch Foods Inc.	United States	681.2
8	Perdue Farms	United States	667.7
9	Sanderson Farms Inc.	United States	622.4
10	Industrias Bachoco	Mexico	622.0

(*Source*: Clements, 2020)

4.2.2 Indian Scenario

Figure 4.10 shows the contribution of meat production from cattle, buffalo, sheep, goat, pig and poultry in the total meat produced across the country during 2018-19. The diagram shows that nearly fifty percent of meat production is contributed by poultry. buffalo, goat, sheep, pig, and cattle contributes nearly 19, 14, 8, 5 and 4 percent of meat production respectively to the total meat production of the country.

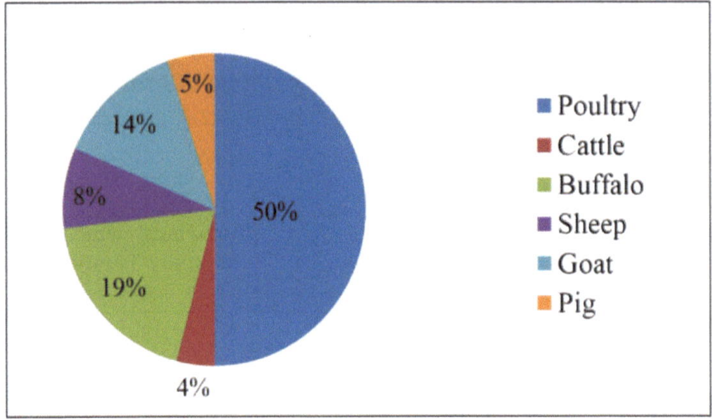

Fig. 4.10: Species wise meat contribution 2018-19

Poultry Meat Production

The total meat production of the country is 8.11 million tonnes. The meat production from poultry is 4.06 million tonnes. The poultry meat production has increased by 7.8 percent over previous year possibly because of rising domestic demand for poultry meat. The growth in the broiler segment is expected to remain strong due to consumer preference for poultry, increasing income levels, and changing food habits. The live market sales of broiler meat still constitute more than 90-95 percent of total volume of sales; the processed chicken meat segment comprises only about 5 percent of total production. Broiler production is mainly concentrated in Maharashtra, Haryana, West Bengal, Tamil Nadu and Andhra Pradesh.

Table 4.17: Meat production and per capita availability

Year	Chicken meat production ('000 tonnes)	Human population (in million nos.)	Per capita availability (kg/annum)
2009-10	2087.35	1170	5.61
2010-11	2193.14	1186	5.41
2011-12	2483.10	1210	4.87
2012-13	2681.60	1212	4.52
2013-14	1916.61	1228	6.41
2014-15	3045.21	1244	4.09
2015-16	3263.81	1260	3.86
2016-17	3463.65	1275	3.68
2017-18	3766.94	1290	3.42
2018-19	4061.79	1305	3.21

(*Source*: BAHS, 2019; BAHFS, 2018; BAHFS, 2017; BAHFS, 2015; BAHFS, 2014)

The broiler poultry production is increase over the time from year 2013-14. It has reached from 1916.61 to 4061.70 thousand tonnes in year 2018-19.

Broiler Poultry- Growth Rate

Table 4.18: Annual growth rate of chicken meat production

Sr.No.	Year	Annual growth rate (%)
1	2011-12	13.22
2	2012-13	8.06
3	2013-14	-28.36
4	2014-15	58.85
5	2015-16	6.89
6	2016-17	6.13
7	2017-18	8.87
8	2018-19	7.83

The growth rate of broiler production is fluctuating over the period. It has registered the growth rate of 7.83 percent in year 2018-19.

Table 4.19: Trends in broiler industry

Parameters	1990	2015
Broiler parents housed (Crores)	0.7	3.5
Broilers placements month (Crores)	5	25
Broiler feed price (Rs/kg)	20	30
Chicken per head (kg)	0.4	2.5
Broiler price/kg live (Rs)	25	65
Broiler integration (Percent)	0	60
Broiler FCR	2.2	1.65
Days to slaughter (2 kg)	48	38
Multi-age group farms (Percent)	90	10
Chicken processing (Percent)	1	7
Antibiotics issue (Percent)	Nil	50

(Source: Kotaiah, 2016)

Table 4.20: Chicken meat production during 2014-15 to 2018-19 of different states(in 000 tonnes)

Sr.No.	States/UTs	2012-13	2013-14	2014-15	2015-16	2016-17	2017-18	2018-19
1	Maharashtra	80.64	143.65	434.37	450.11	517.45	571.20	632.32
2	Haryana	6.47	352.12	367.24	382.45	407.75	440.32	478.63
3	West Bengal	17.57	328.48	338.08	383.80	397.16	437.28	475.42
4	Tamil Nadu	4.25	225.08	346.48	412.15	427.53	440.62	455.51
5	Andhra Pradesh	499.19	133.76	320.99	301.47	317.80	390.06	443.35

Sr.No.	States/UTs	2012-13	2013-14	2014-15	2015-16	2016-17	2017-18	2018-19
6	Uttar Pradesh	6.17	269.67	304.38	334.23	353.49	356.64	359.44
7	Telangana			245.33	262.06	288.00	314.25	336.33
8	Kerala	378.78	49.39	163.60	175.02	188.76	181.97	178.03
9	Karnataka	14.39	81.83	82.61	83.54	87.12	121.34	139.18
10	Punjab	0.56	103.42	108.47	108.08	112.07	114.39	125.03
11	Odisha	328.50	28.54	73.79	74.83	82.37	84.59	98.25
12	Bihar	6.33	28.81	43.15	47.02	53.32	59.38	64.43
13	Jammu & Kashmir	62.72	5.96	18.65	39.47	44.71	48.89	52.50
14	Chhattisgarh	31.39	17.77	27.02	29.39	34.71	38.00	40.29
15	Madhya Pradesh	65.03	16.00	20.39	22.78	26.41	30.79	37.07
16	Tripura	1.56	20.00	21.99	24.48	25.48	29.80	32.08
17	Gujarat	0.48	30.04	30.57	30.80	30.41	30.71	31.13
18	Jharkhand	128.84	2.48	9.56	10.71	12.67	16.52	16.41
19	Rajasthan	7.09	28.40	25.71	22.92	8.40	9.97	10.85
20	Assam	23.73	6.14	7.50	8.00	8.69	9.38	10.73
21	Uttarakhand	0.78	3.63	8.12	8.58	8.86	9.16	9.50
22	Manipur	25.41	6.74	8.50	6.55	7.06	6.69	8.07
23	Puducherry	7.06	7.20	7.22	7.35	7.43	7.36	7.37
24	Meghalaya	334.43	4.56	4.29	4.17	2.61	3.62	4.64
25	A&N Islands	0.00	1.41	4.23	4.28	4.32	4.43	4.55
26	Goa	333.71	3.44	1.18	3.53	2.93	3.49	3.69
27	Mizoram	245.15	1.59	1.66	1.84	2.03	2.04	2.18
28	Nagaland	4.93	0.53	1.08	0.94	0.78	0.51	1.83
29	Himachal Pradesh	7.65	0.45	0.46	0.58	1.05	1.19	1.25
30	Sikkim	6.77	0.78	0.78	3.95	1.36	1.38	0.70
31	Arunachal Pradesh	35.66	0.41	0.13	0.42	0.57	0.59	0.60
32	Lakshadweep	0.23	0.29	0.30	0.68	0.32	0.33	0.34
33	Chandigarh	0.00	0.00	0.00	0.00	0.00	0.05	0.08
34	Daman & Diu	0.00	0.00	0.00	0.00	0.00	0.00	0.00
35	D.& N. Haveli	0.00	0.00	0.00	0.00	0.00	0.00	0.00
36	Delhi	16.12	14.05	17.38	17.37	0.00	0.00	0.00
	India	2681.60	1916.61	3027.83	3263.81	3463.65	3766.94	4061.79

(*Source*: BAHS, 2019; Basic Animal Husbandry and Fisheries Statistics (BAHFS), 2018; BAHFS, 2017; BAHFS, 2015)

Table 4.20 shows that, the leading poultry meat producing states are Maharashtra, Haryana, West Bengal, Tamil Nadu and Andhra Pradesh.

Models of Broiler Farming

A farmer interested in broiler poultry farming has two options:

i. **Non-Contract Broiler Farming (NCBF)**: In this set-up, the farmer has to bear all the expenses, such as Extension Advisory Services from private poultry consultants; procurement of chicks, feed, medicines and vaccines; overhead farm expenses (labour, electricity, water, litter material, farm disinfection, etc.); and transportation. The farmer has to admit all three risks – investment, production and market risks.

ii. **Contract Broiler Farming (CBF)** /Integration: In this case, the integrator provides EAS and inputs such as chicks, feed, medicines and vaccines. The integrator bears the transportation cost, investment (inputs) and marketing risks. The contract farmer provides labour, shed, electricity, water, litter material, and other miscellaneous services or equipment that may be required. Because the major chunk of the expense (working capital) is borne by the integrators, they are the absolute owners of the movable stock (broiler birds) on the farm, and the farmer's role is that of caretaker who gets a predetermined price, which is listed in the contract. This payment to the farmer is linked to various parameters such as the FCR, mortality of birds, etc. A farmer is rewarded for surpassing the set standards and penalized if any of the agreedon criteria is not met. The integrator is also relieved of his biggest threat disease outbreak as his millions of birds are reared at different locations in relatively small numbers by several small farmers.

Table 4.21: Major differences between CBF and NCBF

Parameter	**CBF**	**NCBF**
Land provision (owned/leased)	Farmer	Farmer
Broiler shed and equipment (around Rs. 150/sq. ft., depending on automation level)	Farmer	Farmer
Costs of labor, electricity/fuel, disinfecting shed, litter material	Farmer	Farmer
Manure after liquidation (sale/own consumption), empty feed bags	Farmer	Farmer
Working capital (chicks, feed, medicines, vaccines and veterinary supplies)	Supplied by integrator	Farmer purchases from market
EAS, routine and emergency veterinary services	Provided by integrator freely	Farmer pays poultry consultants

Marketing risk	Integrator lifts the live birds and sells through own outlets/ value addition	Farmer bears the risk
Rearing charges (RC) (incentives/ penalties - for efficiency/high sale rate/high mortality	Integrator pays RC to the farmer for labor, litter, electricity, equipment and shed costs, and also a part of profit	Not applicable
Returns to farmer	Almost fixed	Depend on the market sale rate

(Source: Sasidhar and Suvedi, 2015)

4.2.3 Gujarat state scenario

The estimate of broiler reared in the year 2018-19 is 23472533 compared to previous year's 23261531, showing an increase of 0.91 percent. Total poultry meat production is estimated at 1323.62 metric tonnes from deshi birds, 4645.10 metric tonnes from improved layers and 25162.56 metric tonnes from broiler birds. Gujarat has 8 registered slaughter houses.

Table 4.22: Number of registered slaughter houses and number of broiler birds slaughtered in Gujarat state for the year-2018-19 (in Nos.)

Sr.No.	Name of the District	No. of Registered Slaughter Houses	No of Broiler Birds Slaughtered
1	Ahmedabad	1	739771
2	Amreli	0	17489
3	Anand	0	3399481
4	Banaskantha	0	757749
5	Bharuch	0	1204953
6	Bhavnagar	0	221204
7	Dahod	0	244585
8	Dang	0	63540
9	Gandhinagar	0	1142215
10	Jamnagar	0	1047843
11	Junagadh	1	464953
12	Kachchh	0	47792
13	Kheda	0	1998752
14	Mahesana	0	246817
15	Narmada	0	112572
16	Navsari	0	2780006
17	Panchmahals	0	294814
18	Patan	0	138128
19	Porbandar	0	190140
20	Rajkot	1	909806
21	Sabarkantha	0	1600888

22	Surat	2	1527508
23	Surendranagar	1	32583
24	Vadodara	1	2265138
25	Valsad	1	1872919
26	Tapi	0	150887
	Gujarat State	8	23472533

(*Source*: DOAH, 2020)

Table 4.23: Estimated average meat production of poultry, Gujarat state for the year 2018-2019 (in kg)

Sr.No.	Name of the District	Deshi Layer Yield*	Improved Layer Yield*	Broiler Birds Yield*	Meat Prod. of Poultry
1	Ahmedabad	5714	391546	793034	1190294
2	Amreli	3763	0	18748	22511
3	Anand	5641	2425461	3644243	6075345
4	Banaskantha	28426	33512	812307	874245
5	Bharuch	63994	13770	1291710	1369473
6	Bhavnagar	7548	836751	237130	1081430
7	Dahod	143240	0	262195	405436
8	Dang	59150	0	68114	127264
9	Gandhinagar	2712	3059	1224455	1230226
10	Jamnagar	5849	46364	1123288	1175500
11	Junagadh	22209	32897	498430	553536
12	Kachchh	4499	0	51233	55732
13	Kheda	16378	152350	2142662	2311390
14	Mahesana	4783	28814	264588	298185
15	Narmada	43983	0	120677	164661
16	Navsari	113158	147189	2980167	3240514
17	Panchmahals	130118	0	316041	446159
18	Patan	7254	43178	148073	198505
19	Porbandar	547	20486	203830	224863
20	Rajkot	4097	78215	975312	1057624
21	Sabarkantha	34556	12029	1716153	1762738
22	Surat	137019	175090	1637489	1949598
23	Surendranagar	801	0	34929	35731
24	Vadodara	112975	56086	2428228	2597289
25	Valsad	235624	88770	2007769	2332162
26	Tapi	129578	59536	161751	350865
	Gujarat State	1323617	4645102	25162558	31131277

(*Source*: DOAH, 2020)

*(*Average layer bird yield 0.934 kg/bird, Average broiler yield 1.072 kg/bird)*

5

Backyard Poultry Farming (Unorganized Sector)

Backyard farming is an unorganized sub sector of poultry industry. India has nearly 60 percent of its population living in rural areas. However, in the present scenario most of the commercial poultry production is concentrated in urban and semi urban areas due to high demand. Only 25 percent population living in urban area consumed about 75-80 percent of eggs and poultry meat. Non-availability of poultry products and low purchasing power of the rural people devoid them of access to the highly nutritious products like egg and meat, thereby, resulting in malnutrition. Free range and small scale semi commercial back-yard poultry production can be advantageously promoted in rural areas, as the large commercial poultry production continues to be concentrated in urban and semi-urban locations. It can be used as a powerful tool for alleviation of rural poverty, eradication of malnutrition and creation of gainful employment in vast rural areas (Sharma and Chatterjee, 2009; Rajkumar *et al.*, 2010).

The most basic and simple backyard production system involves a few hens and a cockerel is essentially a closed system. Home-produced fertile eggs are hatched to provide replacements, birds feed by scavenging or are provided with household scraps and crop by-products; there are virtually no veterinary inputs and the remaining eggs and meat produced are consumed within the household. Such very simple subsistence poultry production systems are probably quite rare. Producers with even slightly larger flocks, generate cash income from the sale of eggs and birds within the local community. Transactions may take place directly between producers and consumers, but traders and other market intermediaries may be involved, selling on to other sectors of the poultry industry. Village or backyard production systems are widely distributed and exist in both rural and urban areas. It is estimated that today in India, about 18 percent of total poultry output is derived from backyard production.

In areas that are less densely populated by poultry, backyard systems are likely to contribute a larger proportion of total poultry production. In the village or backyard sector, production is generally based on traditional local, native breeds, producing both eggs and meat. In the recent past, improved backyard varieties (like Vanaraja, Gramapriya, Srinidhi, Giriraja *etc.*) developed mostly by public sector and a few by private sector (like Kroiler, Rainbow rooster) are substantially contributing to the total chicken egg and meat production of the country. Furthermore, given the lower opportunity costs of resources and the higher market prices offered for local poultry, backyard systems are likely to yield a positive economic return, despite increasing competition from the commercial sectors.

Registered native chicken breeds and their conservation

A total of twenty native chicken breeds have been recognized and registered as indigenous breeds of chicken in India.

Table 5.1: Registered native chicken breeds

Sr. No.	Breed	Home Tract
1	Ankaleshwar	Gujarat
2	Aseel	Chhattisgarh, Orissa and Andhra Pradesh
3	Busra	Gujarat and Maharashtra
4	Chittagong	Meghalaya and Tripura
5	Danki	Andhra Pradesh
6	Daothigir	Assam
7	Ghagus	Andhra Pradesh and Karnataka
8	Harringhata Black	West Bengal
9	Kadaknath	Madhya Pradesh
10	Kalasthi	Andhra Pradesh
11	Kashmir Favorolla	Jammu and Kashmir
12	Miri	Assam
13	Nicobari	Andaman & Nicobar
14	Punjab Brown	Punjab and Haryana
15	Tellichery	Kerala
16	Mewari	Rajasthan
17	Kaunayen	Manipur
18	Hansli	Odisha
19	Uttara	Uttarakhand
20	PD2 (Vanaraja Female) Line	ICAR-Directorate of Poultry Research, Hyderabad

(*Source*: www.nbagr.res.in)

Table 5.2: Improved breeds for backyard poultry farming

Sr.No	Name of variety	Name of the organization	Purpose
1	Gramapriya	DPR, Hyderabad	Egg
2	Krishna J	JNKVV, Jabalpur	Egg
3	CARI Gold	CARI, Izztnagar (U.P)	Egg
4	CARI Nirbheek	CARI, Izztnagar (U.P)	Egg
5	CARI Shyama	CARI, Izztnagar (U.P)	Egg
6	CARI Hitcari	CARI, Izztnagar (U.P)	Egg
7	CARI Upcari	CARI, Izztnagar (U.P)	Egg
8	Gramalakshmi	KAU, Mannuthy	Egg
9	Kalinga Brown	CPDO, Bhubaneswar	Egg
10	Kaveri	CPDO, Hessarghatta	Egg
11	HH260	CPDO, Hessarghatta	Egg
12	KrishiBro	DPR, Hyderabad	Meat
13	CARI Dhanaraja	CARI, Izatnagar (U.P)	Meat
14	AVM Coloured	AVM Hatechery, Coimbatore	Meat
15	Chabro	CPDO, Hessarghatta	Meat
16	Vanaraja	DPR, Hyderabad	Dual
17	CARI Devendra	CARI, Izatnagar (U.P)	Dual
18	Giriraja	UAS, Banglore	Dual
19	Swrandhara	KVAFS, Hebbal (Karnataka)	Dual
20	Nicorock	CARI, Portblair	Dual
21	Nishibari	CARI, Portblair	Dual
22	Nandanam- 1 & 2	TANUVAS, Cheenai	Dual
23	Gramapriya	KAU, Mannuthy	Dual
24	Gramshree	KAU, Mannuthy	Dual
25	Kuroiler	Kegg Farm, Delhi	Dual
26	SatpudaDeshi	YeshwantAgro Tech, Jalgaon	Dual
27	Assel Cross	AICRP on poultry Breeding, Assam	Dual
28	Deepika	Central Island Agricultural Research Institute, Portblair	Dual
29	Jharsim	AICRP, Ranchi Center	Dual

(*Source*: Sheikh *et. al.*, 2018; Reddy, 2018; www.cari.icar.gov.in; www.farmerjunction.com)

Table 5.3: Backyard breeds suitable for different states

Sr. No.	States	Birds suitable for rearing in the backyard
1	Andaman and Nikobar Island	Nikobari, Gramapriya, Vanaraja
2	Andhra Pradesh	Gramapriya, Vanaraja, Srinidhi(New), Rajashri. Indbro(Pvt.), Kuroiler(Pvt.)
3	Arunachal Pradesh	Chabro, Nirbheek, Kuroiler(Pvt.), Kamarupa(new), Kalinga Brown
4	Assam	Kamarua(new), Kalinga brown, Chabro, Nirbheek, Keroiler (Pvt)
5	Bihar	Jharsim (new), Shipra (Pvt.), Kuroiler(Pvt.)
6	Chandigarh	Chabro, Nirbheek, Kuroiler(Pvt.)
7	Chhattisgharh	Narmadanidhi(new), Saptpuda Desi(Pvt.), Chhabro
8	Dadara & N Haveli	Saptpuda Desi(Pvt.), Chhabro
9	Daman & Diu	Saptpuda Desi(Pvt.), Chhabro
10	Goa	Saptpuda Desi(Pvt.), Chhabro
11	Gujarat	Pratapdhan(new), Chhabro
12	Hariyana	Chabro, Nirbheek, Kuroiler(Pvt.)
13	Himachal Pradesh	Chabro, Nirbheek, Kuroiler(Pvt.)
14	Jammu & Kashmir	Chabro, Nirbheek, Kuroiler(Pvt.)
15	Jharkhand	Jharsim(new), Shipra(Pvt.)
16	Karnataka	Giriraja, Girirani, Swarnadhara
17	Kerala	Nandanam 99, Giriraja, Girirani, Swarnadhara
18	Lakshadweep	Nandanam 99, Giriraja, Girirani, Swarnadhara
19	Madhya Pradesh	Narmadanidhi(new), Saptpuda Desi(Pvt.), Chhabro
20	Maharastra	Saptpuda Desi(Pvt.), Chhabro
21	Manipur	Chabro, Nirbheek, Kuroiler(Pvt.), Kamarupa(new), Kalinga Brown
22	Meghalaya	Chabro, Nirbheek, Kuroiler(Pvt.), Kamarupa(new), Kalinga Brown
23	Mizorum	Chabro, Nirbheek, Kuroiler(Pvt.), Kamarupa(new), Kalinga Brown
24	Nagaland	Chabro, Nirbheek, Kuroiler(Pvt.), Kamarupa(new), Kalinga Brown
25	NCT of Delhi	Chabro, Kuroiler(Pvt.)
26	Odisha	Kalinga Brown
27	Puduchhery	Nanadanam 99, Giriraja, Girirani, Swarandhara
28	Punjab	Chabro, Nirbheek, Kuroiler(Pvt.)
29	Rajasthan	Pratapdhan(new), Chhabro
30	Sikkim	Chabro, Nirbheek, Kuroiler(Pvt.), Kamarupa(new), Kalinga Brown
31	Tamil Nadu	Nanadanam 99
32	Telangana	Gramapriya, Vanaraja, Srinidhi (New), Rajashri
33	Tripura	Chabro, Nirbheek, Kuroiler(Pvt.), Kamarupa(new), Kalinga Brown

Sr. No.	States	Birds suitable for rearing in the backyard
34	Uttar Pradesh	Chabro, Nirbheek
35	Uttarakhand	Chabro, Nirbheek
36	West Bengal	Chabro, Nirbheek, Kuroiler(Pvt.), Kamarupa(new), Kalinga Brown

(*Source*: National Action Plan for Egg & Poultry - 2022 for Doubling Farmer's Income by 2022, 2017)

Government Schemes for Unorganised Sector

a) Rural Backyard Poultry Development (RBPD)

It is a component of National Livestock Mission (NLM), which covers beneficiaries from BPL families to enable them to gain supplementary income and nutritional support. Under RBPD, the chicks/ birds suitable for rearing in the backyard are reared in the mother units up to 4 weeks and are further distributed to the BPL beneficiaries in at least two batches.

b) Innovative Poultry Productivity Project (IPPP): Transform backyard poultry to commercial economic model

IPPP is launched under NLM which is for scaled-up the poultry model from backyard to entrepreneur, up-scaling incremental up to 400-1000 birds. In case of Low-input technology (LIT) birds, these would help in transition and up scaling later to 1,000-2,000 birds for larger commercial scale poultry farming. Similarly, it is also envisaged to introduce smaller scale broilers in rural households for later scaling up to commercial scale and have poultry as a mainstream source of income. Similarly, small scale broiler farming is envisaged to be introduced in cluster approach.

Pilot Intervention	Activity	Milestones (2017-18 to 2021-22)
Innovative Poultry Productivity Project (IPPP) to be implemented on pilot basis in 15 States	To encourage Broiler Rearing by giving 600 broiler chicks in 4 batches	Distribution over four years of 72 lakh broilers in 4 batches of 150 birds each year at intervals of 3 months; This will produce 123 lakh kg meat valued at Rs. 12312 lakh and benefit around 12,000 beneficiaries. Later it will be upscale to about 50,000 landless/ marginal farmers.
	400 Low-Input Technology (LIT) birds in 2 batches with a gap of one and a half years	Distribution over 2 years of LIT birds - 200 in first year and then after 18 months to be repeated twice i.e. over 4 years 48 lakh LIT chicks to be distributed to 12,000 beneficiaries; This will produce 61.20 lakh kg meat and 2880 lakh eggs valued at Rs. 26,280 lakh. Later it will be upscaled to about 50,000 landless/ marginal farmers.

6

Contribution of Indian Poultry Sector in National Economy

Table 6.1 and table 6.2 shows the Gross Value Added (GVA) of poultry sector in Indian economy. The GVA from poultry sector in year 2017-18 at current price was Rs. 32844 Crore and Rs. 101913 for eggs and meat respectively.

Table 6.1: GVA from poultry sector at current prices (Rs. in Crore)

Year	Eggs		Poultry meat		GVA form livestock sector
	Value (Rs. in Crore)	Percentage Share	Value (Rs. in Crore)	Percentage Share	
2011-12	16633	5.08	39583	12.09	327334
2012-13	19690	5.34	47740	12.94	368823
2013-14	22708	5.37	59620	14.10	422733
2014-15	24382	4.78	65313	12.80	510411
2015-16	26657	4.58	74793	12.84	582410
2016-17	29756	4.42	96505	14.34	672829
2017-18	32844	4.33	101913	13.44	758417

(*Source*: BAHS, 2019)

The GVA from poultry sector in year 2017-18 at constant (2011-12) price was Rs. 21876 Crore and Rs. 76924 for eggs and meat respectively.

Table 6.2: GVA from poultry sector at constant (2011-12) prices (Rs. in Crore)

Year	Eggs		Poultry meat		GVA form livestock sector
	Value (Rs. in Crore)	Percentage Share	Value (Rs. in Crore)	Percentage Share	
2011-12	16633	5.08	39583	12.09	327334
2012-13	17364	5.04	42470	12.33	344375
2013-14	18308	5.04	49681	13.67	363558
2014-15	19080	4.89	53120	13.60	390449
2015-16	19829	4.73	60066	14.31	419637
2016-17	20346	4.41	72873	15.80	461171
2017-18	21876	4.43	76924	15.58	493676

(*Source*: BAHS, 2019)

7

Trade Performance of Poultry Sector

7.1 Global

Major poultry products which are traded in world market are live poultry, edible poultry meat, cuts and offals excluding livers, eggs in shells, eggs not in shell, egg yolks, egg powder etc.

Table. 7.1: Major exporters of poultry products in world, 2018

Rank	Exporting Country	Qty. (MT)	Value in (000 USD)	Share (%)
1	Brazil	35,74,847	61,81,517	19.12
2	Netherland	20,16,740	37,44,313	11.58
3	U S A	27,24,641	35,57,668	11.00
4	Poland	12,96,106	28,31,678	8.76
5	Germany	14,12,542	25,17,625	7.79
6	France	7,98,523	16,22,130	5.02
7	Belgium	6,82,926	11,24,793	3.48
8	China P RP	8,56,221	10,17,552	3.15
9	Hungary	2,68,351	9,35,296	2.89
10	Thailand	18,85,552	7,48,853	2.32
36	**India**	**22,44,157**	**67,717**	**0.21**

(*Source*: Agricultural and Processed Food Products Export Development Authority (APEDA), 2019)

The leading exporter in poultry products in the world is Brazil with export value of 61,81,517 (000) USD followed by Netherland and USA with value of 37,44,313 (000) USD and 35,57,668 (000) USD respectively. India is way behind in the exports at 36th rank with share of 0.21 percent in year 2018.

Table. 7.2: Major importers of poultry products in world, 2018

Rank	Importing Country	Qty. (MT)	Value (000 USD)	Share (%)
1	Germany	14,51,901.00	34,19,687.00	10.58
2	Netherland	16,01,615.00	23,29,695.00	7.21
3	U K	5,80,683.00	19,65,946.00	6.08
4	Hong Kong	9,36,322.00	16,39,632.00	5.07
5	France	5,71,557.00	16,17,486.00	5
6	Japan	5,87,513.00	15,06,687.00	4.66

Rank	Importing Country	Qty. (MT)	Value (000 USD)	Share (%)
7	China P RP	5,23,901.00	13,96,008.00	4.32
8	Saudi Arab	6,66,301.00	13,46,778.00	4.17
9	Mexico	10,12,232.00	12,75,687.00	3.95
10	Belgium	8,70,174.00	10,24,817.00	3.17
118	**India**	**7,839.00**	**6,260.00**	**0.02**

(*Source*: APEDA,2019)

Table 7.2 shows major importers of poultry products in the world in 2018. Germany is the major importer with share of 10.58 percent in total import. India's rank in total import is 118th with share of 0.02 percent.

7.2 India

India is exporting more raw material than processed product, which shows that India have less processing capacity and value-addition. Major market for Indian poultry products are Middle East and Asia. Some products like egg powder also exported to Japan and EU. Major exported poultry products are table eggs, egg powder, hatching eggs, SPF eggs, live birds, and poultry meat.

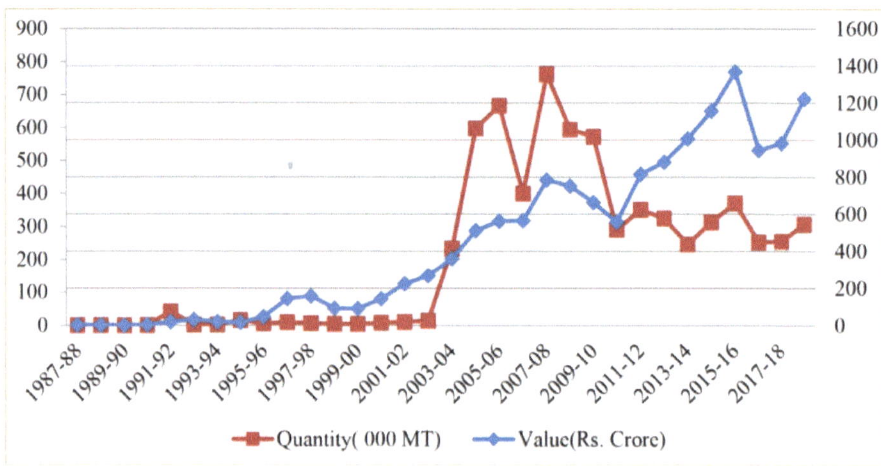

Fig. 7.1: India's export of poultry products over the year in value and volume

It is noted that though the volume of exports was commensurate with the value of exports, it is desirable to have low-volume high-value products to have more profitability.

Poultry products ranked 25th place in terms of total export with contribution of 637.3 Crore and share of 0.5 percent in India's export. Major importing countries of Indian poultry products are Oman, Maldives and Japan which hold share of 35.25, 9.45 and 7.96 percent respectively.

Table 7.3: Major importing countries of Indian poultry products (Quantity in MT and Rs in Crores)

Country	2016-17		2017-18		2018-19		Growth (%) on previous year	Share (%) in 2018-19
	Qty.	Rs.	Qty.	Rs.	Qty.	Rs.		
Oman	2,36,916	159	2,90,261	205	3,27,647	242	18.22	35.25
Maldives	1,11,837	49	1,15,342	52	1,34,318	65	26.04	9.45
Japan	630	19	750	24	1,361	55	125.87	7.96
Vietnam Soc. Rep.	1,633	27	3,034	44	4,562	51	16.44	7.43
Indonesia	1,437	45	1,109	37	1,180	42	12.79	6.15
Netherland	324	8	585	21	762	27	29.97	3.92
Russia	1,388	36	1,052	28	867	25	-10.73	3.59
Nigeria	409	14	430	14	661	24	72.25	3.55
Saudi Arab	4,974	42	636	17	738	22	28.39	3.23
Qatar	0	0	16,465	11	44,616	21	89.87	3.01
Bhutan	795	10	1,545	13	1,567	20	54.64	2.91
Baharain	28,475	31	9,555	10	11,445	17	70.38	2.45
Kuwait	302	1	4,876	10	6,503	13	37.95	1.95
United Arab Emts.	3,716	17	1,283	10	712	10	-1.84	1.48
Germany	568	14	439	12	289	9	-25.62	1.35
Thailand	405	14	318	11	364	8	-19.59	1.24
Taiwan	202	6	141	5	161	6	25.28	0.85
Philippines	130	4	165	5	144	5	5.92	0.8
Iran	7,557	6	306	4	786	5	38.16	0.71
Nepal	54	0	86	2	316	5	173.74	0.68
Other	46,975	27	5,589	18	5,986	14		2.02
Total	4,48,725	530	4,53,967	552	5,44,985	687	24.48	100

(*Source*: APEDA, 2019)

8

Marketing Stucture of Poultry Sector

The greater the distance between producer and consumer, the more complex is the marketing organization required to ensure that eggs reach consumers in the form, place and time desired. Producers may decide to market their produce directly to consumers - direct marketing - or may choose from a variety of marketing organizations that make up a marketing channel.

8.1 Direct Marketing

Direct marketing includes the following methods of selling:

- Sales from the farm (farm gate)
- Door-to-door sales
- Producers' markets
- Sales to local retail shops

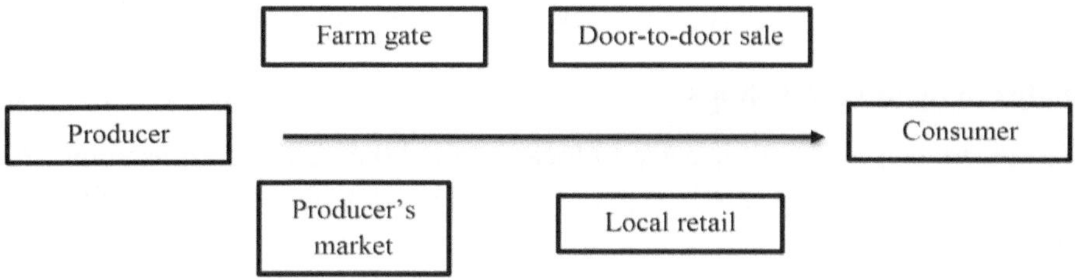

Fig. 8.1: Direct marketing

Egg producers who are situated a short distance from consumers may be able to practise direct marketing. Before choosing to sell their products directly to consumers, however, they must evaluate two main factors:

- Time : Producers who choose direct marketing have less time for production activities.
- Cost : The costs involved in direct marketing.

There are four main ways to carry out direct marketing.

Sales from the farm

Producers may be able to sell eggs directly from the farm (farm gate). This, however, will depend on whether consumers are able and willing to go to the producer's facilities. The main advantage of farm-gate selling is that the producer may be able to obtain a market price for eggs without incurring marketing costs. The main advantage for the consumers is that eggs will be fresh with little or no quality loss.

Door-to-door sales/street hawking

Some consumers prefer that eggs be brought directly to their door. This means that the producer must spend time on marketing; however, consumers may appreciate the service and be willing to pay a good price. Furthermore, the producer can take orders directly from consumers and carry only what he/she is assured will be bought. Eggs may also be sold on the street.

Producers' markets

Usually the producer simply occupies a stall in a public marketplace and offers his/her produce for sale. Eggs are commonly displayed in baskets and often differentiated by weight/size and colour. Sales in producers' markets permit a farmer to make direct contact with consumers who are not able to go to the production facilities. The main disadvantage of using such markets is that, towards the end of the day, the producer may have to either reduce his prices sharply to dispose of remaining stock or carry it back to the farm.

Sales to local retail shops

Producers can also sell directly to local retail shops. This requires some sort of agreement between the two parties regarding constant supply, quality and payment methods.

In some cases it may be possible for producers to sell directly to institutional consumers such as hotels, restaurants, schools and hospitals. This type of direct marketing, however, requires negotiation, which may result in a written contract of the duties and obligations of both parties. It also requires continual interaction over time between producer and buyer, a standard egg quality agreement and a constant supply. The producer must carefully evaluate the issues involved including the regular production and transport of large quantities of eggs.

8.2 Organized Marketing Channel

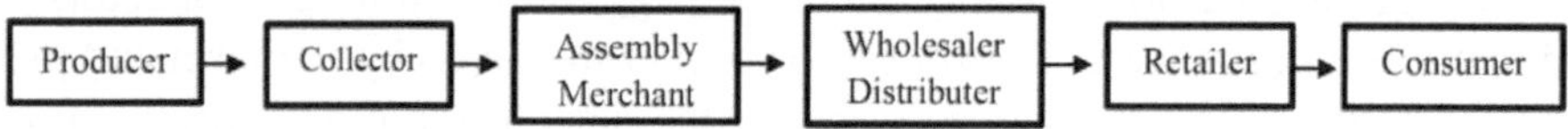

Fig. 8.2: Organized marketing channel

A marketing channel is composed of a set of separate but interdependent organizations involved in the process of making a product available to consumers. The use of a marketing channel is convenient particularly when the producer does not have the time or financial means to carry out direct marketing. Intermediaries are usually able to make the product widely available and accessible because they are specialized and have experience and contacts. They also have a better understanding of the egg market. Intermediaries take the risks involved in marketing and also pay for the produce immediately.

Marketing intermediaries

Collectors

Collectors undertake the initial work of assembling eggs from various producers or local country markets. They operate either on a commission basis or by purchasing on their own account. Where the quantity of eggs collected at each stop is small and frequent, this system is often the most economic. Collectors may be itinerant merchants, producers themselves, assembly merchants, wholesalers or their agents, or retailers.

Assembly merchants

Assembly merchants may be divided into the following categories: local assembly market; independent processor-packer; and, cooperative processor-packer.

Local assembly market

In a typical local assembly market, a private firm, a producers' cooperative or a municipality provides an enclosed space for the use of sellers. Sales may take place by public auction or by private negotiation, subject to rules such as those on quality and payment arrangements. Auctioning requires the eggs to be graded and possibly presented in standardized containers, marked with identifying names or symbols. The local assembly market may provide cold storage facilities for the convenience of market users.

Independent processor-packer

This type of enterprise usually purchases eggs either through collectors or directly from producers. The processor-packer may pass by the farm and pick up the eggs or the producer may deliver the eggs to the processing facilities where they are graded and packed. Usually eggs are sold to wholesalers; however, they are also sold directly to retailers and institutional consumers such as hotels, restaurants and hospitals.

Cooperative processor-packer

The same type of enterprise may be set up and run by a cooperative association of producers. The main advantage is that the business is run by and for those who use it, rather than by those who own it. Cooperatives can obtain financing, provide extra competition to independent processor-packers and provide an alternative to established intermediaries.

Before forming a cooperative, producers should carefully evaluate:

- Market for eggs
- Problems in existing marketing channels and how to remedy them
- Degree of know-how that producers have in marketing
- Rules and regulations
- Legal status
- Availability of finances
- Staffing requirements
- Appropriate geographic location

Wholesale distributor

Wholesaling includes all the activities involved in selling goods to those who buy for resale or for business use. The main function of the wholesale distributor is to balance supplies against retail requirements and to take the initiative of bringing produce from areas where it is plentiful and cheap to those where it is relatively scarce and expensive. Wholesalers usually have a good knowledge of the market, access to the best information on trends and prospects and working capital to carry business risks as required.

Wholesalers usually obtain eggs from central wholesale markets, assembly merchants, collectors and local country markets; however, in some instances they go directly to the producers. Eggs may be purchased directly or accepted for sale on a commission basis. Many wholesalers have their own storage facilities. Wholesale distributors may engage specialized transport agencies to transport eggs or operate such services on their own account.

Central wholesale markets

Central wholesale markets receive shipments from large farms and from country markets, and constitute a supply source where wholesalers and retailers can obtain the various types of produce they need. General wholesale markets sell many different products, including eggs. Because it is the focus point of many smaller markets and also the point of contact for suppliers to important groups of consumers, a central market is usually the primary price-making mechanism for the production areas it serves. In this way it balances demand and supply.

Retailer

In urban areas, egg sales are made through retailers. Four types of retailers usually carry eggs in their shops:

- Poultry shops where only eggs and poultry are sold
- Food shops specializing in eggs, poultry, cheese, butter, meat and fish
- General food shops and supermarkets selling all kinds of foods and household goods
- Meat markets where all types of meat are sold and eggs are also offered for sale

In some instances retailers buy eggs directly from the producer and may have their own process-packing facilities. (Source: FAO, 2003)

8.2. Producer's Association

The National Egg Coordination Committee (NECC), which has a membership of more than 25,000 farmers and traders, is the largest association of poultry farmers in the world. Its genesis goes back to 1981, when the Indian poultry industry was going through unprecedented crisis. The control trade of middlemen forced down the prices down and farmers were being paid less than their production cost. The business had become economically unviable because the feed costs had more than double and the egg price remained static at 35 paisa. So, the farmers had stopped the operations. Determined to do something, the late Dr. B.V. Rao, along with a group of farmers, started a mass movement – they travelled across the country holding meetings with farmers and traders. Their objective was to unite poultry farmers from all over India, and see that they get better prices by eliminating intermediaries from the trade. Thus, NECC was born. Since then, NECC has played a significant role in the betterment of poultry farmers, and the egg industry in general, through its various programmes such as market intervention, pricesupport operations, egg promotion campaigns and consumer education.

The manifold activities of NECC include: To decide upon a reasonable price for eggs which ensures a fair return to the farmers, decent margins to the middleman and a fair price to the customer.

- Price declaration.
- To monitor the egg stock levels in different production centres.
- Manage stock levels and regulate the movement of stocks from surplus to deficit regions, in order to maintain a balance between demand and supply.
- Market intervention through Agrocorpex India Limited.
- To organize and unite poultry farmers across the country.
- To create a dependable distribution network so that eggs could reach every household in every village.
- To generate employment by encouraging people to take up egg farming and egg trading.
- To promote exports and develop export markets
- To make available the technology and information for increased production of eggs.
- To get government support and financial aid from banks for various schemes in rural India.
- Advertise with the objective of educating the customer.
- Undertake a powerful egg promotion campaign to counter the myths about the egg and communicate it's benefits. This would help increase the level of consumption of eggs.
- Market research, identification and its development.
- Preparation and submission of position papers to the government on issue affecting the industry.

NECC is a completely voluntary body created by farmers, and runs on cooperative spirit. It makes no profits and subsists mainly on contributions from its members. (Mehta and Nambiar, 2007; www.e2necc.com)

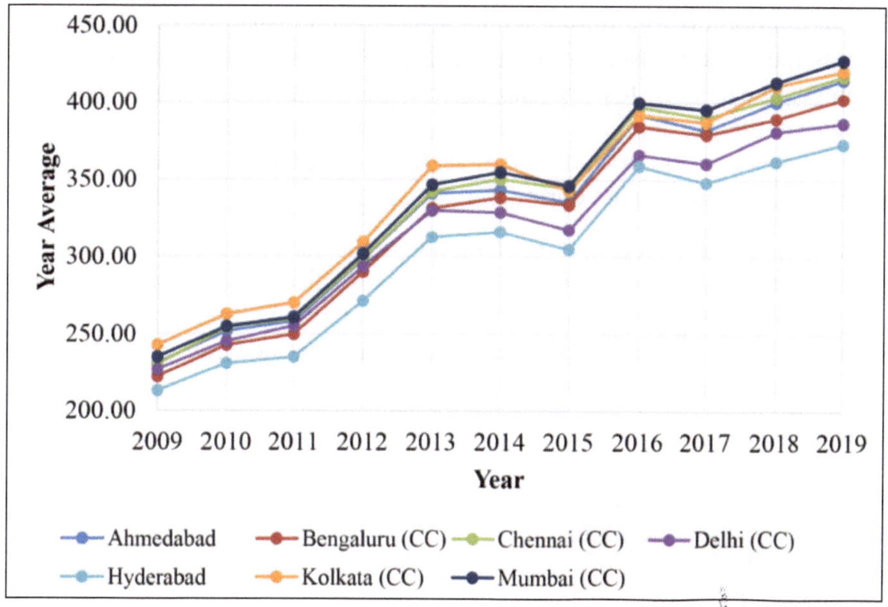

Fig. 8.3: Last 11 years price trend of 100 eggs

Figure 8.3 revealed that the average egg prices had grown significantly from 2009

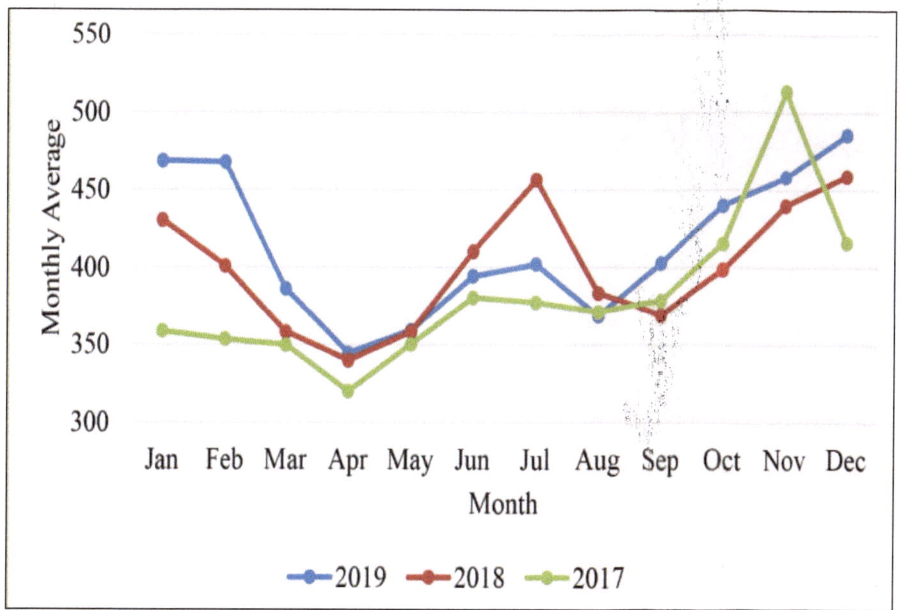

Fig. 8.4: Monthly price of 100 eggs in Ahmedabad market

The consumption of egg during winter season is high and this results in high prices in the market. Also, the demand is high in the months of November and December due to many festivals like Bakrid, Christmas and New Year, and this attributes to the rise in prices. The lowest price was observed during the month of April, due to lower demand for egg in all the market centers of India and the reason includes hot climate during months of March, April and May.

In the broiler sector, there is no national organization that looks after the producers' interests. No doubt, some regional organizations have emerged and are trying to organize farmers, but the broiler marketing is largely in the hands of big traders and commission agents. In general, intermediaries are vital links between producers and consumers.

(Mehta and Nambiar, 2007)

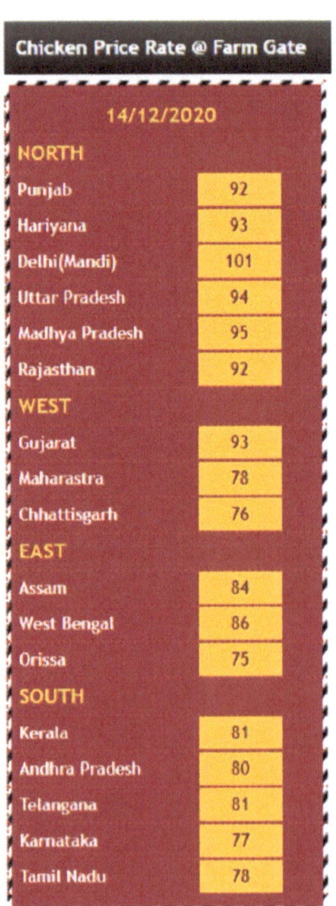

Chicken Price Rate @ Farm Gate	
14/12/2020	
NORTH	
Punjab	92
Hariyana	93
Delhi(Mandi)	101
Uttar Pradesh	94
Madhya Pradesh	95
Rajasthan	92
WEST	
Gujarat	93
Maharastra	78
Chhattisgarh	76
EAST	
Assam	84
West Bengal	86
Orissa	75
SOUTH	
Kerala	81
Andhra Pradesh	80
Telangana	81
Karnataka	77
Tamil Nadu	78

Fig. 8.5: Chicken prices disseminated by All India Poultry Development & Services Pvt. Ltd.

9

Growth Drivers and Emerging Trends

a) Large Unpenetrated Market

According to the sample registration system (SRS) baseline survey, 2014 released by the registrar general of India, 71 percent of Indians over the age of 15 are non-vegetarian.

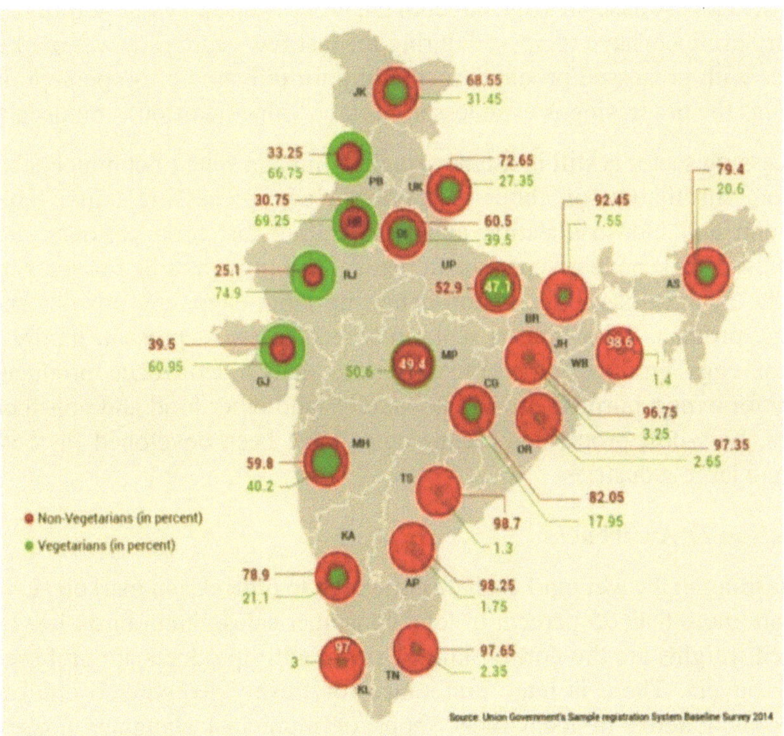

b) Young Growing Population and Nutritional Security

India as a one of the major young population country in the world (27.4%) according to FAO, OECD 2018 data there is a huge need to address the nutritional security of the people with higher protein diet. Thus, we have high requirement of protein to feed country's population in up- coming years.

c) Per Capita Consumption & Income

The annual per capita consumption of broiler meat and eggs for India is far below then recommended consumption of 180 eggs and 10.8 kg poultry meat per person per annum by Indian Council of Medical Research.

The increase in per capita disposable income has led to an overall increase in food consumption, particularly protein in the form of meat and eggs. (McKisney and company Report, 2013). The study conducted by Law *et al.* (2019) suggested that in India the consumer preference has changed and the cereals are now substitute of animal products rather than a complementary product.

d) Poultry Processing and Value Addition

This is still at a very nascent stage but both the processing and value addition of the poultry products have increased during the last few years. The wet market dominates with processed products accounting for only about 5-6 percept. In case of eggs the processing is even lesser. Further, value-addition is miniscule.

Egg processing sector is still in infancy stage in India in spite of commendable production. Installation of about half-a-dozen egg processing units, rapid urbanization and industrialization and proliferating fast food parlours, etc. over the last decade have given some impetus to the growth of egg processing sector. The country has, thus, begun exporting table eggs, egg powder and frozen egg products on a limited scale in recent years. At present, hardly 5 percent of eggs produced are processed into dehydrated/frozen products, primarily for export purpose or used in bakeries and other food and non-food industries. Low-cost processing technologies have been developed for both cottage and large industries.

e) Education & Awareness

India is leading in the wet market share compared to other Asian markets. Live broilers are more than 95 percent of total consumer sales. Small birds 1.8-2.0 kg dressed weights are the norm. Skinless raw poultry products are preferred by many buyers. There is huge preference for freshly slaughtered chicken which is slaughtered in local meat shops or municipal slaughter houses. The reasons behind this preference may be many. Indian consumer is price conscious. Industry must come forward to create awareness about processed products. This will not only help in the improvement of production lines but will also promote consumption of healthy, safe and hygienic meat products among Indian population. Chilled poultry is said to be gaining more rapidly than frozen, but both are a very small share of the total market.

f) Changed Consumer Preference

The consumer preference has changed in recent time. Consumers prefer to buy their meat from branded and hygienic retail meat shop instead of buying from the local butchery shop. The consumers want the products free from hormones, steroids or antibiotics and any other growth promoters. The consumers prefer to order online via e-commerce websites and apps and other marketplace like Dunzo, Swiggy, Zomato etc. Consumers demand increase towards ready to eat/cook products. This leads to the market in more organized in urban sector with the spotlight on safety and hygiene standard and the more customer centric business models, supply chain remodelling and efficiencies driving value creation is expected in the sector.

g) Regulatory Framework

Relevant Acts promulgated by DADF, Government of India

i. The Prevention & Control of Infectious and Contagious Disease in Animals Act, 2009 to regulate disease transmission from one state to other with the objectives:

ii. Indian Veterinary Council Act, 1984 regulates Veterinary Practice and Education

iii. Importation of Livestock and Livestock products are regulated by the Livestock Importation Act, 1898 **Other Acts, Rules & Regulation**

i. Food Safety & Standards Act, 2006 ii. Quality Control of Food Products of Animal Origin (Export-oriented) iii. Residue Monitoring Plan (export-oriented) iv. Agreement on Sanitary and Phyto-sanitary Measures (Global Trade-Oriented)

v. Bureau of Indian Standards (BIS) & ISO 22000:2005 vi. The Prevention of Cruelty to Animals Act, 1960 vii. The Export (Quality Control and Inspection) ACT, 1963

10

SWOT Analysis of Poultry Sector

Strengths

- Poultry farming generates early and regular income and has shorter generation interval.
- Poultry and poultry products constitute an important component of human diet. The consumption is also increasing at a rapid rate due to low fat content, easy availability and cost effectiveness.
- Poultry is the least cost alternative food source next to fish only and produces more animal protein from the same amount of feed. Two eggs provide 160 calories of energy constituting more than 20 percent of the daily requirement of Proteins, Vitamin A, D & B_{12}, Riboflavin, Folic acid, Pantothenic acid, Phosphorus and Iodine along with fat.
- According to nutritional Advisory committee of India, at least half an egg should be made available to an average individual which workout to be 180 eggs/annum. Poultry farming require less area with high and quick return than any other animal husbandry and agriculture activities.
- Good infrastructure like road, rail, ports, airports, reliable electricity power and easily approachable to major cities of adjoining states.

Opportunities

- Growing demand of egg and poultry meat.
- Land requirement for poultry unit is less.
- Sizable population of unemployed rural/tribal youth and women.
- Rising export potential.

Weaknesses

- Social taboos in adoption of poultry entrepreneurship.
- Price fluctuations and seasonal consumption pattern.

- Highly capital intensive.
- Slow adoption of automation in production system.
- Unorganized market.
- Inadequate cold chain facilities for vaccines and cold storage facilities for poultry products.
- Lack of chicken based food processing industries.

Threats

- Outbreaks of emerging and re-emerging diseases.
- WTO: exposing the local industry to global competition.

11

Challenges and Issues Before Poultry Sector

Poultry sector is expected to play the most crucial role in transforming the nutritional demography of country with ever growing share of protein based cheap human diets. Some of the specific challenges the poultry sector is faced with are as follows:

a) Regional imbalances in poultry production

The commercial layer farming is yet to make a dent in some of the region of country. However, broiler farming is gradually catching up in majority region.

b) Underexploited poultry diversity

Among poultry species, chicken production has already acquired large scale commercial dimensions in some states due to its better efficiency. However, there is a scope for exploitation of other domesticated poultry species.

c) Rising feed cost

The growth in poultry has outpaced the growth in cereal production leading to severe feed shortages and consequent rise in feed cost. Cereal by-products and oilseed residues usually constitute more than 80 percent of poultry diet. Coarse cereals also form the staple diet of millions of marginal farmers and landless labourers. These coarse cereals are the most important and most widely used poultry feed ingredients all over the world. The demand for coarse cereals is continuously increasing at 4 percent per year due to ever increasing population and their use in livestock rations.

The yield of maize grain, the most important ingredient of poultry feed in India is just about 40 percent of the world's average. The consumption and production gap will keep rising due to growth of poultry sector as also due to its increasing industrial use (for production of maize starch and high fructose corn syrup etc.).

Soybean meal is yet another important poultry feed ingredient used as protein source in poultry rations. Instability in its production and exports has resulted in its shortage for the poultry industry leading to its high prices.

Poultry feed accounts for 70 percent of the total cost of poultry production. This has become one of the most serious challenges for the industry owing to growing population, alternative uses and resultant increase in demand for the poultry feed ingredients, hence their escalated prices. Therefore, improving feed conversion efficiency would be crucial to profitability apart from the feed cost itself. Over the past two decades, feed conversion rates for poultry have improved by about 40 percent due to improved productivity and efficient feeding strategies. However, still only 25-35 percent of the nutrients consumed by poultry are utilized. Hence, further understanding of digestive physiology and biochemistry can be expected to improve nutrient utilization efficiency.

d) Poultry health management

The available infrastructure to address the health care aspects of poultry such as accredited disease diagnostic laboratories, disease monitoring and surveillance services and training facilities are inadequate in the state. Moreover, the cost of prophylactics and therapeutics is also on the rise. Therefore, technology driven cost-effective and efficient disease monitoring, diagnosis and combat systems need to be devised to address the health care issues concerning poultry.

e) Emerging and re-emerging poultry diseases: high vulnerability to disease outbreaks

In the past, poultry sector has faced frequent onslaught of newer poultry diseases like bird flu (Avian Influenza) leading to enormous losses to the poultry sector not only in Gujarat but India and globally. The total losses to the Indian poultry sector till 2009 have been estimated to the tune of over Rs. 2200 crore. In addition to this, other existing diseases *viz*. Infectious Bronchitis, Infectious Bursal Disease, Ranikhet Disease, Marek's Disease and Fowl Pox have emerged in more virulent form. Therefore, scientific interventions are urgently needed to curb the menace of such emerging poultry diseases in the state as well as effective control measures against already existing major poultry diseases.

In recent times, the poultry industry in India hit hard because of nationwide lockdown to stop the rapid spread of COVID-19 virus. This lock-down had disrupted the entire supply chain. Before COVID-19 the prices for broiler was about Rs. 80 per kg and Rs. 4 for egg the price dropped to almost no value like Rs. 6 per kg and Rs. 1-1.50 per egg. As a result, the projected loss of the industry was about Rs 25000 crore. (Shukla & Bhattacharyya, 2020).

f) Poultry waste disposal and environmental concerns

The magnitude of poultry wastes is constantly on increase due to growth of the poultry industry. The problem of waste disposal is all the more grave due to concentration of poultry in some well-defined pockets or geographical boundaries. There is a need to devise cost-effective ways and means for proper disposal of wastes arising from hatchery and poultry manure to minimize environmental pollution and for putting them to alternative efficient use. Some of the alternative uses of poultry waste are production of manure or bio-fertilizers (vermi-compost) etc. Promotion of cost-effective methods of waste disposal has to be taken up to entice the commercial sector for putting the same into practice.

g) Declining share of backyard/small scale poultry

Rural poultry production constitutes important component of agricultural economy in State, small poultry holders are practically capable of contributing more significantly to alleviate malnutrition, poverty and unemployment. Gujarat requires both mass production as well as production by masses to cater both its rural and urban population. Hence, fund and R&D support is critical for spread and popularization of small scale poultry amongst farming community having less than 2.0 ha. of land holding.

h) Climate change and associated stresses

Impact of climate change is likely to be observed on a higher scale in poultry sector as poultry is more sensitive to changes in temperature, humidity etc. leading to loss of productivity. Therefore, technology driven systems need to be evolved to counter such climate associated threats. Hence, strategies are required to be evolved for meeting these challenges.

i) Poultry marketing infrastructure

Marketing of poultry products is the major issue faced by the industry. In the absence of orderly marketing network, sufficient regulated markets, lack of adequate cold-chain etc., the wholesale prices of poultry products suffer violent fluctuations and often become un-remunerative, due to cyclic boom-and-bust phenomena. The poultry marketing is largely in the hands of commission agents and private traders. Procurement and distribution in remote places receive low priority. Fragmented and remote rural markets also restrict reach of commercial poultry products to the far flung rural areas. Strong marketing network covering the entire state is needed to set the industry free from the clutches of middlemen.

j) World trade and markets

The traditional channels of international trade in poultry have also been distorted owing to frequent outbreaks of deadly poultry diseases like Avian Influenza and COVID.

Limited acceptance of processed poultry products in the domestic markets is yet constraint for establishment of processing units and further investments in this area. Wet-marketing of broilers is still preferred and is widely prevalent in the Country in the absence of general awareness about food safety and quality, and statutory provisions to restrict the same. This is the primary reason for almost dismal share (about 0.7%) of the Country in the global poultry trade.

k) Institutional and capital constraints

The available miniscule public funded institutional support is far from adequate for the mammoth poultry sector. Support for Poultry Science education and R&D is meager in the country. Therefore, there is an urgent need to establish Poultry Extension and Research Institute (PERI) in the country. Moreover, there is an urgent need of Central Poultry Disease Diagnostic laboratory, Mobile Poultry Health Monitoring Units and establishment of Regional Poultry Farmer's Training Centers.

The facilities of micro credit to backyard poultry units are needed to promote poultry production by the masses in the State.

l) Human resource needs

Growing poultry sector also requires trained manpower not only to man the commercial establishments but also to support the required R&D in sync with ever evolving scientific needs. It has been estimated that the highly skilled technical manpower requirement of the poultry sector will almost double by 2050, at the present rate of outturn and the present capacity of the educational and training institutions. Besides, the sector would also witness growth in skilled and semi-skilled manpower requirement at least at 5 percent per year for specific and general operations concerning poultry production and processing. Therefore, developing and sustaining the required capacity building infrastructure to meet the ever growing manpower demand of the poultry sector will be a challenge before the State.

12

Nutritional Value of Poultry Products

12.1 Nutritional Value of Egg

The egg is one of the most complete and versatile foods available. It consists of approximately 10 percent shell, 58 percent white and 32 percent yolk. Neither the colour of the shell nor that of the yolk affects the egg's nutritive value. The average egg provides approximately 313 kilojoules of energy, of which 80 percent comes from the yolk. The nutritive content of an average large egg (containing 50 g of edible egg) includes, 6.3 gram protein, 0.6 gram carbohydrates and 5.0 gram fat (this includes 0.21 g cholesterol).

Egg protein is of high quality and is easily digestible. Almost all of the fat in the egg is found in the yolk and is easily digested. Eggs contain every vitamin except vitamin C. They are particularly high in vitamins A, D, and B12, and also contain B1 and riboflavin. Provided that laying hens are supplemented according to the Optimum Vitamin Nutrition concept (see chapter 'Optimum vitamin nutrition of laying hens'), eggs are an important vehicle to complement the essential vitamin supply to the human population.

Eggs are a good source of iron and phosphorus and also supply calcium, copper, iodine, magnesium, manganese, potassium, sodium, zinc, chloride and sulphur. All these minerals are present as organic chelates, highly bioavailable, in the edible part of the egg. (Source: www.thepoultrysite.com)

Table 12.1: Nutritive values of one egg (60g, edible portion 53g) and in whole egg (in 100g)

Constituents	**Unit**	**Per egg (53 g)[a]**	**Per 100 g[a]**
Protein	G	6.8	12.9
Carbohydrates	G	0.4	0.7
Fat	G	5.9	11.1
Essential fatty acids	G	0.7	1.3
n-3 fatty acids	G	0.2	0.4
Minerals			
Sodium	Mg	80	140
Potassium	Mg	80	150
Calcium	Mg	30	56
Phosphorus	Mg	115	216

Constituents	**Unit**	**Per egg (53 g)** [a]	**Per 100 g**[a]
Magnesium	Mg	6.4	12.1
Iron	Mg	1.1	2.1
Fluoride	Mg	0.74	1.4
Iodine	Mg	0.006	0.011
Selenium	Mg	0.013	0.0245
Vitamins			
Vitamin A[e]	Mg	0.15	24.5[d]
Vitamin D	Ug	1.54	2.9
Vitamin E	Mg	1.1	2.0
Vitamin K	Ug	25	48
Vitamin B1	Mg	0.05	0.1
Vitamin B2	Mg	0.16	0.30
Vitamin B6	Mg	0.06	0.12
Vitamin B12	Ug	1.06	2.0
Folic acid/Folate	Ug	34	65
Niacin [f]	Mg	1.6	3.1
Biotin	Ug	13.25	25.0
Pantothenic acid	Mg	0.85	1.6

(*Source*: Sreenivasaiah, 2006)

12.2 Nutritional Value of Poultry Meat

Poultry meat (chicken) is a good source of protein and vitamins and minerals, such as iron, selenium, zinc, and B vitamins. It is also one of the main sources of vitamin B12. It has several advantages as half of the fat from chicken meat is made up of the desirable monounsaturated fats, and only one-third of the less healthy saturated fats. There are much higher proportions of saturated fats in most cuts of red meat, which also vary considerably in total fat. Chicken meat is therefore seen as a healthy meat. Chicken meat does not contain the trans-fats that contribute to coronary heart disease. Poultry meat is rich in the omega-3 fats and is an important provider of the essential polyunsaturated fatty acids (PUFAs), especially the omega (n)-3 fatty acids. Scavenging chickens are a particularly good source because of their varied diet. Poultry meat can be enriched with several of the important dietary nutrients like Selenium whose deficiency is becoming more widespread in humans because soils are becoming depleted and the foods grown on them are therefore lower in selenium.

(*Source*: National Action Plan for Egg & Poultry -2022 for Doubling Farmer's Income by 2022, 2017)

Table 12.2: Composition of meat – Gross (g/100 g edible portion)

Nutrient	Broiler	Turkey	Goose	Duck
Water	65.99	70.40	49.66	48.50
Protein	18.60	20.42	15.86	11.49
Total lipids	15.06	8.02	33.62	39.34
Carbohydrates	Nil	Nil	Nil	Nil
Fiber	Nil	Nil	Nil	Nil
Ash	0.80	0.88	0.87	0.68
Energy, MJ	0.90	0.67	1.55	1.69

(*Source*: Sreenivasaiah, 2006)

Table 12.3: Composition of meat- Vitamins (per 100 g edible portion)

Nutrient (Vitamin)	Broiler	Turkey	Goose	Duck
A, Retinol equivalent	41	2	51	17
C, mg	1.60	Nil	2.80	Nil
B1, mg	0.06	0.06	0.20	0.08
B2, mg	0.12	0.16	0.21	0.24
Niacin, mg	6.80	4.08	3.93	3.61
Pantothenic acid, mg	0.91	0.81	0.95	Nil
B6, mg	0.35	0.41	0.19	0.39
Folic acid, µg	6.00	8.00	13.00	4.00
B12, µg	0.31	0.40	0.25	Nil
NA- Data not available				

(*Source*: Sreenivasaiah, 2006)

Table 12.4: Composition of meat- Minerals (mg/100 g edible portion)

Nutrient (Minerals)	Broiler	Turkey	Goose	Duck
Calcium	11.00	15.00	11.00	12.00
Iron	0.90	1.43	2.40	2.50
Magnesium	20.00	22.00	15.00	18.00
Phosphorus	147.00	178.00	139.00	234.00
Potassium	189.00	266.00	209.00	308.00
Sodium	70.00	65.00	63.00	73.00
Zinc	1.31	2.20	1.36	NA
Copper	0.48	0.10	0.24	0.27
Manganese	0.02	0.02	NA	NA
NA- Data not available				

(*Source*: Sreenivasaiah, 2006)

13

Impact of Covid-19 on Poultry Sector

Agriculture and allied sectors have adversely hit by the COVID-19 scare. The rumors of poultry birds likely the carrier of the virus circulated in social media had led to reduced demand of the chicken meat in several parts of the country in the month of February 2020 even before India reported the first case of COVID-19. The poultry industry in India hit hard because of nationwide lockdown to stop the rapid spread of COVID-19 virus. This lock-down had disrupted the entire supply chain. Before COVID-19 the prices for broiler was about Rs. 80 per kg and Rs. 4 for egg the price dropped to almost no value like Rs. 6 per kg and Rs. 1-1.50 per egg. As a result, the projected loss of the industry was about Rs 25000 crore. (Shukla & Bhattacharyya, 2020).

According to industry sources, the poultry industry which had witnessed steady growth rate in the last two decades because of rising consumer demand for protein rich food especially but, it has incurred huge losses since the beginning of the 2020. The loss incurred by Indian poultry industry is mainly attributed to sharp decline in demand because of disruption of supply chain during lock down. The financial condition of all the stakeholders in the poultry value chain – farmers, feed suppliers and retailers had become risky. The drop in demand and supply chain disruption especially hit the smaller farmers who had limited resources. Thus, many farmers went for 'contract farming' offered by many large poultry players.

To bring back the poultry sector into some short of normal operations, both the Central as well as the State Government provided policy support through declaring supply of poultry products under essential services, ensuring huddle-free interstate transport of poultry produce. The clarification issued by different government agencies and various poultry associations that eating chickens is quite safe, could convince the consumers to a large extent. The poultry industry in India hit hard because of nation-wide lock-down to stop the rapid spread of COVID19 virus. This lock-down had disrupted the entire supply chain.

The situation changed sharply since June 2020 mainly because of rising demand of poultry meat and eggs as doctors advised people to take protein rich food for improving immunity against the COVID-19 virus. As a majority of the working population continued to Work from Home (WFH) mode, the domestic chicken consumption has seen sharp rise. So, when the restrictions were removed, the demand for hygienic and quality poultry products grew sharply leading to a sharp spike in sales of online retail players.

Many new online retail players with their dedicated sourcing as well as modernized processing facilities offered quality poultry meat and egg at the doorstep of consumers. Even demand for eggs has been robust. Many who used to consume vegetarian food have commenced consuming poultry meat and eggs. The consumer demand for poultry meat and eggs started picking up from June and post Navratras & Onam festivals witnessed a sharp spike. The demand for poultry meat and eggs have been rising along with a rise in farm gate prices. The onset of winter months also pushes up the demand for poultry meat and eggs. By observing the opportunities in the market, many poultry players have set up new processing plants and the robust demand in the coming months would definitely see the poultry industry operating at a level witnessed prior to COVID19 emergence in the global scene.

Key aspects which Indian poultry industry need to adopt for creating a robust supply chain and creating strong consumer confidence in the poultry product in the postCOVID 19 phase

- Poultry meat is primarily sold in the fresh markets, as consumers prefer to buy live poultry and get it dressed in their presence. The fresh chicken is sold by small establishments. In the Post-COVID19 phase, the poultry industry should focus on ensuring a Standard Operating Procedure (SOP) for these small chicken meat sellers in maintaining hygiene in the establishment so the consumer confidence in the product is strengthened.
- The industry must focus on promotion of processing for which the existing transportation and cold storage facilities have to be revamped so that seasonal fluctuations in the meat prices could be curbed.
- The processing would also integrate the industry with the online retailers of the meat products.
- The poultry industry must focus on creating consumer confidence through use of social media as well as various other media like print and TV, where benefits of eating chicken could be promoted. • Social media rumours should be monitored and dealt with for creating consumer confidence (Thaper,2020).

14

Conclusions

a) **Transformation towards Commercial Agro:** The poultry sector in India has experienced a revolutionary shift in structure and operation, which has led its transformation from a simple backyard activity to a major commercial agro based industry over a period of decades.

b) **Layer Farming:** The production of eggs has increased from 1.83 billion numbers in 1950-51 to 103.32 billion numbers in year 2018-19. The per capita availability reached at 79 eggs per annum in the year 2018-19 from 5 eggs per annum in year 1950-51. Andhra Pradesh, Tami Nadu and Telangana contributes about 55 percent share in total egg production.

c) **Broiler Farming:** Chicken meat contributes to 50 percent share in total meat production in year 2018-19 with the production of 4.06 million tonnes production. Broiler production is mainly concentrated in Maharashtra, Haryana, West Bengal, Tamil Nadu and Andhra Pradesh. Broiler farming is mainly done through contract broiler farming. In that the integrator provides inputs such as chicks, feed, medicines and vaccines. The contract farmer provides labour, shed, electricity, water, litter material, and other miscellaneous services or equipment that may be required. The integrator bears the transportation cost, investment and marketing risks.

d) **Role of Backyard Farming:** The backyard poultry farming is contributing 18 percent of total poultry production. It is an unorganized sector in which the birds are reared by the rural people for home consumption. In backyard sector production is generally based on traditional local, native breeds producing both egg and meat. In the recent past, improved backyard varieties developed by public and private sectors are Vanaraja, Gramapriya, Srinidhi, Giriraa, Kroiler, Rainbow rooster etc. which are substantially contributing to the total chicken egg and meat production of the country.

e) **Contribution from Gujarat:** Total egg production of Gujarat for the year 2018-19 was 18544 lakh and meat production of poultry was 31131 tonnes.

f) **Key Contribution to Livestock Sector:** Poultry sector contributes Rs. 1347.57 billion in total output of livestock sector which hold 12.91 percent share. Poultry products ranked 25th place in terms of total export with contribution of 637.3 crore and share of 0.5 percent in India's export. Major importing countries of Indian poultry products are Oman, Maldives and Japan which hold share of 35.25, 9.45 and 7.96 percent respectively.

g) **A Steady Income:** Poultry farming generates early and regular income and has shorter generation interval.

h) **Health Benefit:** The poultry products are the cheapest source of protein, and it can play the major role for national food security.

i) **A Raising Demand:** The demand of egg and poultry meat is rising due to changing in the food habit of the people. However, some of the challenges faced by the sector are, higher input cost (mainly feed cost), price fluctuations and seasonal consumption pattern, lack of marketing infrastructure, less value addition, Inadequate cold chain facilities for vaccines and cold storage facilities for poultry products, Outbreaks of emerging and re-emerging diseases.

References

Chatterjee, R. N., & Rajkumar, U. (2015). An overview of poultry production in India. *Indian Journal of Animal Health*, *54*(2), 89-108.(Retrieved from: https:// fdocuments.in/reader/full/an-overview-of-poultry-production-in-india-poultryproduction-systems-into-four)

Clements,M.(2020,October),Topworldbroiler,eggrankingfor2020.PoultryInternational,59(10), 4-42.(Retrieved from: https://www.poultryinternationaldigital.com/*poultryinternational/* october_2020/MobilePagedReplica. action?pm=2&folio=32#pg34)

Delgado, C., Narrod, C.A., & Tiongco, M. M. (2003). Policy, technical and environmental determinants and implications of the scaling-up of livestock production in four fast-growing developing countries: A synthesis. *International Food Policy Research Institute*, *188*. (Retrieved from: https://www.researchgate. net/publication/265079481_Implications_of_the_Scaling-up_of_Livestock_Production_in_a_Group_of_Fast-growing_Developing_Countries)

Directorate of Animal Husbandry. (2020). 36th Survey report on estimates of major livestock product for the year 2018-2019 Gujarat state. (Retrieved from: https:// doah.gujarat.gov.in/Images/animalhusbandary/pdf/36th-Survey-Report-of-MLP. pdf)

Food and Agriculture Organization. (2003). Egg marketing-a guide for the production and sale of eggs. *FAO Agricultural Services Bulletin* 150, 29-51. (Retrieved from: http://www.fao.org/3/Y4628E/y4628e06.htm#bm06)

Government of India (2014). Basic Animal Husbandry and Fisheries Statistics. (Retrieved from:https://dahd.nic.in/sites/default/filess/BAHS%20%28Basic%20Animal%20Husbandry%20Statistics-2019%29_0.pdf)

Government of India. (2015). Basic Animal Husbandry and Fisheries Statistics. (Retrieved from: https://dahd.nic.in/sites/default/filess/BAH_%26_FS_Book.pdf)

Government of India. (2017). Basic Animal Husbandry and Fisheries Statistics. (Retrieved from: https://dahd.nic.in/sites/default/filess/Basic%20Animal%20Husbandry%20 and%20 Fisheries%20Statistics%202017%20%28English%20version%29_5.pdf) Government of India. (2018). Basic Animal Husbandry and Fisheries Statistics. (Retrieved from: https://dahd.nic.in/sites/default/filess/BAHS-2016%20Updated%20on%20 16.08.16_0.pdf)

Government of India. (2019). Basic Animal Husbandry Statistics. (Retrieved from: https://dahd.nic.in/sites/default/filess/BAHS%20%28Basic%20Animal%20 Husbandry%20 Statistics-2019%29_0.pdf)

Government of India. (2017). National Action Plan for Egg & Poultry -2022 for Doubling Farmer's Income by 2022. (Retrieved from: http://www.indiaenvironmentportal. org.in/files/file/Seeking%20Comments%20on%20National%20Action%20 Plan-%20Poultry -%202022.pdf)

Hendrix Genetics. (2020). Nutrition Guide. Boxmeer, Netherlands: Leentfaar E. (Retrieved from:https://layinghens.hendrix-genetics.com/documents/883/Nutrition_Guide_English_vs3.pdf)

Intodia, V. (2016). Poultry and Poultry Products Annual. *Global Agricultural Information Network.* (Retrieved from: https://apps.fas.usda.gov/newgainapi/ api/report/ downloadreportbyfilename?filename=Poultry%20and%20Poultry%20 Products%20 Annual%202016_New%20Delhi_India_12-1-2016.pdf)

Karthikeyan, R., & Nedunchezhian, V. R. (2014). An analysis of price trends and its behavioural patterns of the Indian poultry market with reference to egg. *African Journal of Agricultural Research*, *9*(1), 8-13. (Retrieved from: https:// academicjournals.org/ journal/AJAR/article-full-text-pdf/0C8F9B242528)

Khan, L. A. (2019, August 14). Poultry sector clarifies 'myths' around consumption of broiler chicken. *The Hindu.* (Retrieved from: https://www.thehindu.com/ news/national/ karnataka/poultry-sector-clarifies-myths-around-consumption-ofbroiler-chicken/ article29095820.ece)

Kotaiah, T. (2016, March 10). Poultry Production in India - The Current Scenario. *FNB News.* (Retrieved from: http://fnbnews.com/Poultry/poultry-production-in-india-the-current-scenario-38620)

Law, C., Fraser, I., & Piracha, M. (2019). Nutrition transition and changing food preferences in India. *Journal of Agricultural Economics,* 71(1), 118-143. (Retrieved from: https:// onlinelibrary.wiley.com/doi/full/10.1111/1477-9552.12322)

Mckisny and Company (2013). India as an agriculture and high value food powerhouse: A new vision for 2030, Food and Agriculture Integrated Development Action 3. (Retrieved from: https://www.mckinsey.com/~/media/mckinsey/featured%20 insights/ india/india%20as%20an%20agriculture%20and%20high%20value%20food%20 powerhouse/india%20as%20an%20agriculture%20and%20high%20 value%20food % 20powerhouse%20a%20new%20vision%20for%202030_ report.ashx)

Mehta, R., & Nambiar, R. G. The poultry industry in India. (Retrieved from: http://www. fao. org/ag/againfo/home/events/bangkok2007/docs/part1/1_5.pdf)

Organisation for Economic Co-operation and Development. (2018). *OECD-FAO agricultural outlook 2018-2027.* (Retrieved from: http://www.fao.org/3/I9166EN/ i9166en.pdf)

Rajkumar, U., Rao, S. R., & Sharma, R. P. (2010). Backyard Poultry Farming changing the face of rural and tribal livelihoods. *Indian Farming, 60*(2).

Reddy, J. (2018, November 19) Kuroiler Chicken Breed Profile. *Agri farming.* (Retrieved from: www.agrifarming.in/kuroiler-chicken-breed-profile-andcharacteristics#:~:text=%20 Physical%20Characteristics%20of%20Kuroiler%20Chciekn%20Breed%3A%20 ,3.5%20kg%20%287.7%20lb%29%20and%20 females...%20More%20)

Research and markets (2019). India's Poultry Processing Market 2018-2023 - Market projected to Reach INR 107.6 Billion by 2023. (Retrieved from: https://www. globenewswire. com/news-release/2019/11/26/1952555/0/en/India-s-PoultryProcessing-Market-2018-2023-Market-Projected-to-Reach-INR-107-6-Billionby-2023.html)

Sasidhar, P. V. K., & Suvedi, M. (2015). Integrated contract broiler farming: an evaluation case study in India. *Feed the Future.* (Retrieved from: https://meas.illinois.edu/ wp-content/ uploads/2015/04/MEAS-EVAL-2015-Broiler-India-short-SasidharSuvedi-July-2015. pdf)

Sharma, R. P., & Chatterjee, R. N. (2009). Backyard poultry farming and rural food security. *Indian Farming*, *59*(36-37), 48.

Sheikh, I. U., Nissa, S. S., Zaffer, B., Akand, A. H., Bulbul, K. H., Hasin, D., Hussain I & Hussain, S. A. (2018). Propagation of backyard poultry farming for nutritional security in rural areas. *International Journal of Veterinary Sciences and Animal Husbandry*,

3(4), 03-06. (Retrieved from: https://www.veterinarypaper.com/ pdf/2018/vol3issue4/ PartA/3-3-21-133.pdf)

Shukla, P. K. & Bhattacharyya, A. (2020). Impact of COVID-19 on Indian Poultry Sector. *The Poultry Punch.* (Retrieved from:https://www.thepoultrypunch.com/2020/05/ impact-of-COVID-19-on-indian-poultry-sector .)

Sreenivasaiah, P. V. (2006). Scientific Poultry Production, A unique encyclopaedia (3rd ed.). *Luncknow, UP. : International Book distributing Co.*

Thaper, R. (2020). Robust Consumption Growth in Last Six Month Helps Poultry Industry Back on a Growth Path in The Post-Covid19 Scenario. *The Poultry Punch.* (Retrieved from: https://thepoultrypunch.com/2020/12/robust-consumptiongrowth-in-last-six-month-helps-poultry-industry-back-on-a-growth-path-in-thepost-covid19-scenario/)

Web References Retrieved

Agricultural and Processed Food Products Export Development Authority (n.d) agriexchange. apeda.gov.in/

All India Poultry Development and Services Pvt. Ltd. (n.d.) http://vencobbchicken. com/

Central Avian Research Institute (n.d) cari.icar.gov.in/varietiesdeve.php

National Bureau of Animal Genetic Resources(n.d) nbagr.res.in/regchi.html

National Egg Coordination Committee (n.d) www.e2necc.com/home/index

Food and Agriculture Organization Corporate Statistical Database (n.d) www.fao. org/faostat/ en/

The Organisation for Economic Co-operation and Development (n.d) www.data. oecd.org

www.indianmirror.com/indian-industries/2019/poultry-2019.html

www.farmerjunction.com/poultry-breeds-available-india/

www.thepoultrysite.com/publications/egg-quality-handbook/4/the-nutritivevalue-of-the-egg#:~:text=Neither%20the%20colour%20of%20the%20shell%20nor%20that,g%20of %20edible%20egg%29%20includes%3A%206.3%20g%20protein

Index